Wellness In a Toxic World

Martin S Gildea DC CFMP

INTENDED USE STATEMENT

All of the material written in this book is intended for informational purposed only and is not to be used in any way to diagnose, treat, cure, or prevent any disease. The book attempts to emphasize environmentally and nutritionally significant information. Healthy choice suggestions are made to support health maintenance

MEDICAL DISCLAIMER:
Individuals should always consult their health care provider before administering any suggestions made in this book. The contents of this book should not be misinterpreted as a claim or representation in which any product mentioned or procedure constitutes a cure-palliative or ameliorative. All procedures discussed therein along with any nutritional protocols should be considered as alternative or adjunctive to other accepted conventional procedure deemed necessary by the attending licensed physician. The author of this information cannot be held responsible for interpretation of this information for any unintentional misleading omissions of the information. There are no nutritional compounds in this book meant to replace established, medical conventional approaches-especially in serious life threatening diseases or emergencies. None of the contents of this book have been evaluated by the Food and Drug Administration. The fact that an organization or website is referred to in this work as a citation and/or a potential source for further information does not mean that the author endorses the information the organization or website may provide or recommendations they may make. Further, readers should be aware that the internet websites listed in this work may have changed or disappeared between when this book was written and when it was read.

Wellness in a Toxic World

Copyright © 2016 Martin S Gildea DC CFMP

All rights reserved.

No portion of this book, except for brief review, may be reproduced, stored in a retrieval system or transmitted in any form or by other means-electronic, mechanical, photocopying, recording, or otherwise –without the written permission of the author.

ISBN: 9781508838227
Library of Congress Number:

DEDICATION

For my father Professor Martin M. Gildea.

CONTENTS

1	A Toxic Soup	7-18
2	Preferred Lab Tests	21-38
3	The American Diet: Poor Nutrition/Wrong Recommendations	41-61
4	Essential Oils	63-76
5	Nutritional Supplements	79-88
6	Energy Medicine	91-101
7	FCT	103-113
8	PEMF	115-127
9	Nature's Gem Gone Awry: The Immune System	129-133
10	What To Do Next: Applying All Of This To Life	135-156
	Recipes	159-170
	Gluten Free	171-180

ACKNOWLEDGMENTS

I would like to acknowledge my mother and my eldest daughter for all of their hard work in editing this book. I would also like to thank The Johnson Group for continued inspiration which led to the writing of this, my second book.

Introduction

A lot has happened since my last book two years ago; some memorable things like my daughter's college graduation and one unforgettable sad one, the death of my father aged 80 on my 49th birthday. Although he had regular colonoscopies for all of the previously required years, his stage four colon cancer diagnosis was given in April and he was dead in six weeks. Fifteen years ago, he was diagnosed with Melanoma In Situ and had yearly cursory examinations of the skin that found no further problems. Although my mother questioned over the years whether they ordered any internal scans to rule out metastasis, the answer was always no. Following the advice from Sirius radio's world renowned cardiologists, he continued the statin drugs which reduced his total cholesterol levels to what functional medicine practitioners call gravely low levels of 105; a dangerous level for the cancer to cells to proliferate. I must state that there are other methods that could possibly discover cancer or other degenerative disease before there are overt symptoms; <u>functional and energy medicine are at the top of the list</u>. A non- traditional approach to managing chronic conditions by treating each patient individually, it seeks to identify and find the root cause of disease, and views the body as one integrated system. This approach can be extremely valuable for those who have not received the answers or improved their overall state of health through traditional medicine. I continue to ask why the state of Americans' health, compared to other countries, is so inferior. If the old nutritional recommendations were so effective: low fat, seven servings of grains and cow's milk, margarine, unsaturated meats and artificial sweeteners- the SAD (standard American diet), then why have we not become healthier? Why has our infant mortality gone up year after year? **It is time for people to wake up and realize that the whole nutritional system has to be revamped. Until that time, each of us must fend for ourselves in terms of guidelines.**

As I discussed in my previous book, *Health; A Common Sensible*

Approach, we also live in a toxic world of dangerous chemicals and extremely high electromagnetic frequencies all around us at all times including, dirty electricity, silver dental amalgam fillings, fluorescent lights, contaminated fish, and processed foods in our diets. Short of living in the wilderness, it is extremely hard to avoid all of these detrimental effects. More emphasis must be placed on these dangers so that early precautions could be taken. Countless studies from vested interests like the cell phone companies, argue that the phones and their towers are safe just like big Pharma promoting the success of dangerous drugs, many of which are taken off the market. We need to explore the subject from a non-monetarily motivated, more objective eye.

In my office, I explain to a patient what lab tests they should have done to consider how this toxic soup is adversely affecting their health. In addition to the usual blood and urine tests, I also often order hair analysis and or genetic testing, that provides necessary information about a person's susceptibility to certain conditions. After analyzing all of this information, I recommend what therapies and products they need which can make a huge improvement in their quality of life. This could be a godsend for those not getting any better who "have tried everything."

One energy approach I use in my office is Essential oils, an area that my wife Becky, a certified HHP (holistic healthcare practitioner), and I decided to incorporate into our practice. Along with the oils, which complement our other therapies, and get amazing results, I will recommend additional supplements. Although I discussed supplements in detail, in my last book, because innovations are always occurring, I may choose other supplements with superior ingredients that work more efficiently.

To address the toxic soup, other vital forms of energy medicine therapies are needed to both become and remain healthy. Currently, I am incorporating more of this into my treatment tool box if you will. While it seems to be an esoteric subject, there is a plethora of scientific evidence to support it in the field of biophysics, rooted in Einstein's theory on quantum physics.

There are many other forms of energy medicine we use in this office, such as Reiki- in which Becky has advanced training , QRA, FCT (field control therapy) and PEMF (pulsed electromagnetic frequency) which better address and eliminate toxins, exercise cells, and balance energies.

Finally, as in the last book, I will put it all together by summarizing what you can do so that you and your family have the best chance to live a long healthy and productive life up to your genetic potential.

1. A Toxic Soup

We live in a toxic soup. There are over 80,000 toxic chemicals commercially produced in the United States today. Since many have been developed after World War ll, the long term health effects have not been adequately investigated. In order to be produced, these toxic chemicals have to be listed that they are safe in a "low dose." The truth is, however, that many of these chemicals are extremely harmful at very low doses. For example, the herbicide 2,4 ST is harmful in parts per trillion; there are **no** herbicides without dangerous side effects. Another example is liver enzymes. Many patients will tell me their family doctor will periodically check their liver enzymes to make sure the statin drugs or the long term prednisone are not "raising their liver enzymes to dangerous levels." However, unless naturally generated by the body, the chemical levels should be <u>non-detectible not "low level</u>." There are no safe levels, and one has to weigh risk against benefit. A prime example of this is fluoride in the water supply. View the documentary "Flouridegate" at flouridegate.org. that shows although the government knows the harmful effects of fluoridated water, especially on young children, they fight to protect the policies to enforce its use. Long term low doses have been shown to cause ADD-like symptoms of pregnant female offspring in animal studies. A study published in "Brain Research" revealed that a person drinking only 1 part per million fluoride in water had histologic lesions in the brain similar to neurodegenerative diseases such as Alzheimer's or dementia. Long term low levels were also found to build up in bones and weaken their tensile strength allowing for more hip fractures. Hip fractures are a big problem with the elderly in this country. There also has been a steady increase in immune system disorders in the generations exposed to fluoridation since the 1960s and 1970s.

For those of you on-line, check the link, http://scorecard.godguide.com/. Type your zip code and see how your county stacks up against all others in the US by getting a list of the major top polluters and top chemicals released in your county. There is lead hazard information, a list of the worst toxic waste sites or 'Super fund' sites, and also air quality standards so that you can see how your county's air quality stacks up and how many days of clean air quality per year there is and who the top polluters are. Finally, there are water pollution statistics for your county. I am not a tree hugger against big business here, I am simply trying to show how we are BOMBARDED WITH TOXIC CHEMCIALS WHERE WE LIVE UNLESS WE LIVE OFF GRID OUT IN THE BOONIES. This is a real eye opener for many! I use this information to play detective and find out what toxins patients are exposed to which may be a factor in their case. Many have often lived in different places in their lives, and this would mean possible exposure to many different chemical toxins. Let's take a look at how Cumberland, my county, compares to the rest of the country with toxins and pollution. For total environmental releases we are in the 45% range. For air and water cancer risk however, I live in the one of the most polluted counties, with a risk, of 80-90% compared to the rest of the country. What is even worse is that this study was done in 2002! I am sure fourteen years later, we are dumping more hazardous chemicals into the environment. Check this site out.

Let's look at a day in the life of a typical American, for instance, someone in the suburban area. John Doe wakes up in the morning turns off the electric blanket, reaches for his alarm clock and cell phone, a foot or two away from his bed, all emitting strong electromagnetic fields. He may also have his bed only inches away from an electric outlet or only a few feet from the television- both of which also emit strong (EMFs) electromagnetic fields. He then walks into the bathroom and turns on the energy saving lights emitting a large amount of mercury. He brushes his teeth with fluoride, sodium lauryl sarcosinate, and titanium dioxide filled toothpaste.

He shaves with a foaming shaving cream loaded with propylene glycol found in anti-freeze and brake fluid and the mineral water ingredient which is a petroleum product closing his pores. **(1)** Another harsh component is sodium lauryl sulfate, which strips the lipid layer of the skin away so that his skin cannot hold moisture and is more susceptible to bacteria. A quick shower is loaded with chlorine, a toxic chemical which competes with thyroid hormone. He will also use soap and shampoo containing these same harmful ingredients. Anything that really lathers has the **sodium lauryl sulfate** which is a carcinogen, probably the most dangerous ingredient in skin and hair care products. Both a very highly corrosive and cheap detergent, it is used in the cleaning industry as a degreaser. In the skin industry it is used to remove the lipid layer on the skin surface which protects it from drying out. A serious consequence of using products containing this agent is the inability of skin to regulate moisture, often resulting in skin rashes, hair loss and even infection. Ironically, researchers will then intentionally expose this lipid stripped skin to irritants to see what substance will heal the skin. Thus this chemical is the most efficient skin irritant used for conducting experiments! Our typical American man uses his after shave lotion or cologne containing 85% petroleum and would have to be hauled away in a has mat suit as a hazardous waste material. At breakfast there may be more mercury light bulbs and a microwavable pastry with about thirty ingredients. He does not drink any water, but has coffee with an artificial creamer or even skim milk and two teaspoons of white sugar. (I really went into detail about all of the adverse effects of the typical hygiene products used by most people in in my book *Health: A Common Sensible Approach*. I refer you to Chapter five, "A toxic Brew" for a more in depth discussion). He drives to work in a hybrid electric car emitting a huge amount of electromagnetic radiation. Even all non- hybrid gas burning cars emit EMFs due to their having a built in on board computer. In fact, all modern cars emit EMFs to some degree. While driving to work he has a few cigarettes. At work, if in an office, he sits under fluorescent lights loaded with mercury. Sitting at his desk he uses a cordless phone emitting even greater amounts of EMFs than cell phones. All the while he is sitting in a "wireless" internet zone meaning more EMFs. Lunch usually entails going to a restaurant for a sub or pizza, highly processed foods cooked in junk canola oils really devoid of any high quality nutrition. Caffeine loaded Pepsi or Coke is ordered with no water. As I said in the first book, it takes 32 ounces of water to process only 8 ounces of caffeine. You cannot expect the kidneys, which have to filter 2000 liters of blood per day, to function without adequate amounts of salt and water. I can honestly say that 80% of Americans this country are chronically partially dehydrated. Many people tell me they do not "like the taste of water"? They feel if it is in their tea, coffee or soda, that is good enough. **WRONG!!!!!!!!!!!!!!!! When you do not drink enough water your kidneys and adrenals will not function properly.** Most tap water, however, is loaded with the chemicals fluoride and chlorine, both of which are toxic to humans. These toxic chemicals compete with iodine needed to make thyroid hormone which runs the body! He smokes a few cigarettes while at lunch and again while working and on the way home.

After eight hours in this environment, he drives home. He sits under more lights, maybe uses the microwave again and has almost no or very little plain water. Notice that he did not have any vegetables other than the iceberg lettuce on his sub for lunch. No green leafy vegetables means no protection from the toxic soup surrounding him. Finally, after supper he watches television while surfing on his phone or on the computer with Wi-Fi and has more cigarettes: by the end of the day, he has had about one pack or so. Cigarettes contain about 4,000 chemicals. Currently about 20% of Americans smoke. The number one cause of preventable death in the US according to the CDC (centers of disease control.), is cigarettes. Remarkably, this number of smokers has been on the decline over the past few years: however last year nearly 500,000 or one in five deaths were from smoking.

Sometime that evening he meets his girlfriend and gives her a ride to the nail salon. Here she gets her nails done, also a toxic process. Sitting there he notices that it is very hard to breath because of the toxic ammonia smell. He is not hallucinating about that. I remember just walking by the nail salon at a local mall and gasping for air! Nail polish is loaded with toxins,: in fact it contains the infamous concoction known as "the toxic trio," consisting of dibutyl phthalate (DPB), formaldehyde, and toluene. These chemicals are endocrine (hormone secreting glands) disruptors and carcinogens. The problem with many chemicals, as with drugs, is that they produce the desired effect very quickly. In other words, if you want a hardy smooth nail finish (toluene) that will not chip or peel, and you want it to last (formaldehyde) you will have to increase your toxic load. It is hard to find anything natural that will exactly duplicate this. DPB has been linked to lifelong reproductive impairments in male rats: toluene is implicated in anemia and liver damage and formaldehyde is a skin, eye, and respiratory irritant and known carcinogen having been specifically associated with leukemia. In addition to the patrons, one must consider the 121,000 registered nail technicians many of whom are young Asian women, constantly exposed to these toxins 7 days a week. Almost 13,000 chemicals are used in the cosmetic industry and only about 10% have been evaluated for safety. The FDA has the authority to regulate harmful chemicals in cosmetics and other beauty products but does not use it. In 2006 some of the large cosmetic companies announced that they were going to go "three free." However, six years later in 2012 California's Department of Toxic Substances revealed that some products claiming to be non- toxic and even "three free" still contained some or all of the toxic trio. Another announcement claimed that the next generation of nail polishes were going to be "5 free," removing the toxic trio and two other toxic chemicals formaldehyde resin and camphor. The formaldehyde resin is a skin allergen known to cause dermatitis and can off gas some formaldehyde. Synthetic camphor, a scented chemical causing dizziness and headaches when inhaled especially in large doses, is even a larger concern for the nail techs. One solution is to watch the video on YouTube, "How to Buff Your Nails." You can create a nice smooth sheen by buffing nails without using any polish, and they will naturally get stronger and maybe even chip resistant due to the increased circulation. Since nail polish and nail products have been the fastest growing segment of the beauty industry.; Americans spend almost 800 million dollars a year on it! Next our John Doe goes home, falls asleep and repeats the same routine.

Now we must also consider where the power lines come into his house and office where he works. High frequency voltage transients otherwise known as "dirty electricity," can result from a malfunctioning substation in fairly close proximity to buildings occupied by workers or students. **(2)** Studies by Samuel Milham MD, described in his book *Dirty Electricity* reveals that cancer rates in buildings with dirty electricity are much higher than in normal areas. He found a correlation between the length of employment and an increase in cancer risk. His method consisted of using specific meters that measured the aberrant magnetic fields in these buildings. His findings would then be presented to the supervisor in charge who would usually reject them and hire someone who would find non-threatening results. This frequently happens because of the extreme cost of rectifying dirty electricity, yet another example of profits before health. Because of the frequency of these carcinogenic findings, in his many studies, Dr. Milham came up with his own theory in his book *Diseases of Civilization*. One particular study, the Laquinta Middle School study in California seemed to be the impetus of his theory. He contends that these diseases can also be called diseases of longevity and are a result of nations becoming industrialized. Cancer, Type 2 Diabetes, Osteoporosis, cardiovascular, depression, and Alzheimer's are the diseases he is referring to. Conventional thinking, he states, has poor diet, sedentary lifestyle, substance abuse and lack of social values as the cause. However, citing his Laquinta study again, with its connection to an increase in childhood leukemia, Dr. Milham states that "diseases of civilization might instead be diseases of industrialization." Furthermore, he says that examination of mortality rates in the 1930s and 1940s, from all causes, "provides evidence that residual electrification was responsible for the epidemic of our diseases of civilization in the twentieth century." This warrants further investigation.

Toxic agents such as heavy metals are ubiquitous, especially in today's highly technologically advanced society. Scientists often qualify a metal as heavy if its specific gravity is above 4 or 5 or by atomic weight. I prefer the simple definition that it is a heavy metal if it has a potential toxicity to humans and the environment. Many metals could be categorized by this latter definition if taken in large doses- in fact the same ones that are critical in the normal physiological functions in a healthy person- in normal doses such as zinc, copper and iron. For example zinc is a cofactor in many important enzymatic reactions, and hemoglobin contains iron. I maintain that even though toxic at higher levels, many of the metals such as iron and zinc are really not "toxic heavy metals" and should not be categorized as such. The toxic heavy metals I am referring to are lead, cadmium, aluminum, sliver, titanium, tin, nickel, platinum, arsenic, and especially mercury.

Let me talk about how, through normal activities of daily living, we are constantly exposed to the pernicious effects of heavy metals. Many antiperspirants, cookware, canned goods, antacids, buffered aspirin, table salt, and dental amalgams contain aluminum. Because some toothpastes contain aluminum, it is very important to note that drinking water containing fluoride will increase the absorption of aluminum.

The heavy metal Arsenic is found in tobacco smoke and is implicated in lung cancer. Cadmium, what Dr. Marshall, biochemist from Premier Research Labs, calls "white death," is most commonly found in refined foods, white flour, white salt and white sugar. It is also found in tobacco smoke, canned fruits, sodas, margarine and the burning of coal and petroleum products. Lead is another toxic heavy metal found in almost all older homes containing lead based oil paint, canned food, and contaminated water pipes. Nickel is found in pollution from burning coal and petroleum products, cigarettes, costume jewelry, margarine, electronics/computers and hydrogenated oils- the kind used in almost every restaurant because of the low cost. Silver is found mostly in dental fillings, photographic materials and jewelry.

Mercury is the last toxic element I want to discuss. It's the second most toxic substance next to plutonium! Mercury exposure is mostly from dental fillings, large predatory fish consumption, fluorescent lights, pharmaceuticals, paper and plastic manufacturing materials, fungicide on grains and from vaccinations using thimerosal- a mercury based preservative. One extremely disturbing fact about hair mercury levels and intelligence in elementary school aged children is that they have an inverse relationship.

That the amalgam fillings are so prevalent and so disastrous in their effect on the human host's health is the subject of *It's All In Your Head: The Link between Mercury Amalgams and Illness,* a book by a prominent dentist, Dr. Hal Huggins published in 1993. He argued how the American Dental Association admitted a mere 5% of those with mercury amalgams are reactive to them but concluded this was an insignificant number. When Higgins stated that the 5% were epidemic, the ADA reduced the percentage to 1%. He conducted his own trials consisting of over 7000 patients and found that a startling " 90% demonstrate compromised immune activity with low levels of mercury; thus the "credibility battle between organizational prestige and actual tests on patients." **(2)** Dr. Huggins has several cases of how patients' health severely declined after amalgams were put in and then how their health was restored with their removal. The ADA's response was one of denial. They even suggested that one of his video testimonials was faked.

We must also look at xenobiotics, defined as chemical compounds (drug, pesticide or carcinogens) foreign to a living organism. A common category of xenobiotics is pesticides, most notably glyphosate otherwise known as Round-up. Almost everyone with a yard uses this weed killer at least once per year.

Infectious agents are the next category. This includes parasites, bacteria, fungi, and viruses. The SAD (standard American diet) compromises a person's immune system, paving the way for various microbes and bugs to make a home in the body. Due to most people's lack of HCL (hydrochloric acid) or stomach acid, they lack the first line of defense against parasites in sushi. Everybody presently knows about the bacteria resistant bugs from the overprescribing of antibiotics. It is still a huge factor in the increase of bacterial infections. I must also mention Lyme's disease, caused by a female deer tick's bite., leading to the bacterial infection Borelli burgdorferi. Many medical personnel believe that virally infected people are also very susceptible to bacterial infections: therefore they prescribe "preventative" antibiotics. The ineffectiveness of the flu shot is a perfect example of how conventional medicine thinks the virus can just be killed by making antibodies to a specific threat instead of just trying to build overall natural immunity without shots. There are toxins or pernicious agents which will work together or enhance each other's ability to do more harm. For example, with fungi keep in mind that EMF exposure will facilitate the proliferation of it. A fungal infection will also harbor the heavy metal mercury which will make you more susceptible to EMFs.

It appears the SAD (standard American diet) is never far away from any discussions dealing with substances adversely affecting health. I explained this topic thoroughly in my previous book. I must reiterate some key points. Processed food contains a plethora of chemicals which are hard for the body to process, needlessly expending important resources that would be better used elsewhere. Nitrates for example, are preservatives toxic to the nervous system used in many processed meats such as bacon and sausage. The main abuser in the SAD however, is definitely SUGAR!!! Yes, you read it right. Sugar is metabolic poison in large amounts. Everyone would agree the average American's yearly consumption of 150 pounds per year qualifies as a large amount.

Now let's consider drug and alcohol or substance abuse. Many people drink more than the recommended one to two drinks per day; like sugar, alcohol is metabolic poison in high doses. Many forms of alcohol are high in added sugar also, making it even more toxic to the body. Recreational drugs such as heroin and cocaine really just raise the bar for the most amount of damage done by substance abuse. Drugs and alcohol interfere with your body's natural sleep cycle leading me to the next point; most Americans do not get the right amount of sleep versus the amount of time spent at work.

Continuing with our toxic soup discussion, I must address the conventional medical profession's involvement. As I have said many times, the medical profession really succeeds offering excellent acute care dealing with life threatening situations. I am by no means criticizing them for that. My problem, however, is with other than acute emergency medical treatment. They seem to treat all conditions, including chronic ones, the same. Based on the status of this country's mortality rate and overall worldwide health ranking, my criticism is more than founded. Here we have vaccinations as a child. You can group vaccination discussions with those on abortion and religion today because they are such volatile subjects. We spend more per capita on each person in this country, yet the United States is ranked 33rd in infant mortality rates; contributing to this in large part is living in a toxic world.**(3)** The main reasons for high infant mortality rates, which occurring in developing countries, is due to lack of sanitation giving rise to infection and malnutrition. These two factors do not effect an industrialized nation such as the United States. According to the CDC (centers for disease control and prevention), "The relative position of the United States in comparison to countries with lower infant mortality rates appears to be worsening." **(4)** One key factor seems to be the amount of immunizations countries require a child less than one year of age to have. Of the 34 counties ranked above the United States for IMR (infant mortality rate), the top five countries require 12 vaccines - the least amount, while the

United States requires 26 - the highest amount! A recent study was done using a linear regression to find the correlation between the vaccinations doses countries routinely give their infants and their IMR. "These findings demonstrate a counter intuitive relationship: *nations that require more vaccine doses tend to have high infant mortality rates."* **(5)**

Let us look at the top ten prescribed drugs in the United States. According to many authors this list has not changed much in recent years. Coming in at number one is Synthroid or synthetic thyroid hormone. Patients who have lost the ability to produce their own thyroid hormone, will be dependent on an outside source, either natural or more commonly a drug usually for the rest of their life. According to my research on the thyroid, there are over 40 million woman who have a thyroid problem but do not know it due to improper testing and test result interpretation by their physician. Some side effects of Synthroid are heart palpitations and insomnia. When the drug is given the patient has more energy but sometimes this will interfere with the ability to fall asleep. Not to worry however, many doctors will just prescribe Ambien or some other sleep aide. Ambien increases sleep receptor sensitivity in the brain to the neurotransmitter G.A.B.A. by a factor of seven! Talk about zoning out on the spot. In fact, Ambien is also known as the date rape drug. Next, we also have the number two currently highest prescribed drug in the nation is Crestor. The cholesterol tropic is very controversial. Every time you watch the evening news there are cholesterol lowering drug commercials. Recently, however, even conventional medicine seems to be questioning the cholesterol guidelines that have been in place since the seventies. In my last book, I quoted an article written by Dr. Dwight Lundell who operated on thousands of hearts and saw the damage to the arteries the "low fat, low cholesterol diet" had done. **In his conclusion he admitted "that the medical profession really increased instead of deceased heart disease with those faulty recommendations leaving the country in a health crisis."** The antacid Nexium is next. Most people don't produce enough stomach acid instead of too much. The SAD causes food to putrify in the gut which forms lactic acid that will push the undigested food and itself up into the esophagus causing reflux like symptoms. Lactic acid will burn like hydrochloric acid, but it won't digest food. Nexium can cause side effects due to its interference with normal digestion. The body will not absorb Vit B12, calcium or magnesium properly without sufficient levels of stomach acid; without these three, long term use of Nexium may result in such disease processes such as Osteoporosis, chronic diarrhea and seizures. Ventolin is next, also known as albuterol used for bronchospasm or breathing difficulties. Side effects are chest pain with a fast pounding uneven heartbeat, low potassium and dangerously high blood pressure. The number 5 most prescribed drug in 2014 is Advair Diskus, another inhaler for treating asthma that can also be used for certain patients to treat long term chronic obstructive pulmonary disease (COPD). The most common side effects is dizziness; by dilating vessels, blood pressure will drop and affect the body's ability to keep blood in the brain against gravity when the person bends forward.

Diovan is the sixth most prescribed drug on this list, prescribed for high blood pressure. Diarrhea, joint pain and fatigue are the most common side effects. Remember, however, there is no disease called "high blood pressure;" this is actually a condition or result of something else going on in your body. Contrary to the drug company's advertisement, a pill does not just lower your blood pressure making everything ok. High blood pressure could be the result of anything from heavy metal toxicity to mineral imbalance. Next we have the drug Lantus Solostar, a cartridge system that delivers a long lasting form of the hormone insulin to regulate blood sugar levels. Side effects are a lower than normal blood sugar. Number eight on the list is Cymbalta, prescribed for major depression disorders, fibromyalgia and general anxiety. Most Americans, as I stated above, lack sufficient stomach acid to completely digest their foods which then get dumped into the small intestine in a less digested state than desired. This plays havoc with the normal neurotransmitter synthesis- 85% of which takes place in the gut. Actually enabling the gut to function properly can alleviate your depression. Vyvanese is the ninth drug prescribed mostly to young children for attention deficit hyperactivity disorder (ADHD). The most common side effects include insomnia, loss of appetite, and headaches. The loss of appetite reinforces the relationship between the gut and the brain; any drug introduced into the brain chemistry inadvertently will affect not only the brain but also the gut. Last on the list of most prescribed drugs in the United States is Lyrica. indicated for treating seizures, nerve pain from diabetes and fibromyalgia. There are over thirty common side effects from this drug incredibly listed as "not serious" from dizziness to chest pain? **These ten most prescribed drugs** in the United States accounted for 147.6 MILLION MONTHLY PRESCRIPTIONS from July 2013- June 2014!!

Let's look at the top ten best selling drugs. First we have Abilify, an antipsychotic drug used to treat many types of mental illness. Common side effects are dizziness, nausea and vomiting, fatigue, drooling, weight gain, blurred vision and sleep disruption. Teenagers taking this drug, are prone suicidal tendencies. From 7/13-6/14 this drug made $7.1 billion. Humira, next on the list., used to treat two kinds of inflammatory arthritides such as Rheumatoid and Psoriatic. An immune system suppressor, it increases the body's chances of developing a more severe chronic disease or cancer. Common side effects, therefore, are more like allergic reactions- from redness and irritated skin at injection site to headaches and stomach pain. Furthermore, a very serious concern is the possibility of a life threatening anaphylactic reaction. This drug made $6.3 billion 7/13-6/14.

Both Nexium, number three and Crestor number four, the cholesterol lowering drug, accounted for $6.3 and $5.6 billion in sales respectively. Next is Enbrel, number five, prescribed for symptoms related to autoimmune disorders in which the body attacks itself. Like Humira, Enbrel suppresses the immune system and is a tumor necrosis factor (TNF) inhibitor, a substance in the body which reacts by causing inflammation crucial for combating chronic diseases such as cancer. For example, when cancer cells threaten the body, the TNF must try to stop them. **The class of drugs such as Enbrel and Humira will stop all TNF from doing its job leaving an unprotected body susceptible to a serious disease**. Advair Diskus is another drug on the two lists; it brought in a paltry $5 billion. Number seven is Solvaldi, an anti-viral drug which keeps hepatitis C cells from multiplying, and made $4.4 billion. Number eight Remicade is another TNF inhibitor used to treat inflammatory conditions such as Rheumatoid and psoriatic arthritis, Chrohn's and ulcerative colitis for example. Another immune suppressor, Remicade, robs the body's ability to protect itself in the long run; it made $4.3 billion. Lantus Solostar, number nine on the list., the last common drug on the two lists made $3.8 billion from 7/13-6/14. The last drug on the list of top sales is Neulasta, containing a man- made form of protein that manufactures white blood cells in a chemotherapy patient. A serious concern is allergic reactions because it is a synthetic protein, that earned 3.6 billion from 7/13-6/14. **The total from these ten top grossing drugs between 7/13-6/14 is $51 .5 BILLION DOLLARS!!!!!!** I must emphatically remind you to remember that all drugs, aside from side effects, have the ability to leave a residue behind in the body that can continue to be problematic.

Considering the multitude of tests performed on the uninformed public for chronic conditions there are too many routine re-orthopedic, re-x-rays, dental x-rays, and CAT scans with or without contrast media done to warrant their justification. **I am referring to chronic conditions here not any tests needed for life saving hospital emergency visits**. These diagnostic tests leave behind the toxic residue just mentioned which can become problematic many years later. Some of my patients, over the years, were barely able to carry their old heavy x-rays; they had so many!

The United States' philosophy differs greatly from Europe's on setting standards for food and environmental safety. The EU's (European Union) management of chemical and environmental protection policies is based on the precautionary principle that "aims at ensuring a higher level of environmental protection through preventative decision making." On the other hand, the US Federal government's approach to chemical management sets the standard far too high for proof of harm that must be demonstrated before any regulatory action is taken. Here is a list of ten substances readily available in this country but banned in Europe because of their toxicity:

1. **Most GMO foods** such as high fructose corn syrup.
2. **All antibiotics and related drugs fed to livestock** for growth promotion purposes such as bovine growth hormone.
3. **22 pesticides used on crops.**
4. **Chickens washed in chlorine.** All chickens exported from the united states are washed in chlorine and therefore, not allowed in Europe.
5. **Different standards for approving food contact products with chemicals in them.** Plastic bottles for milk or water must undergo proven safety tests by the manufacturer or they are banned. Biphenyl A (BPA) in baby bottles is banned.
6. **Synthetic food colors** such as Red 40, Yellow 5, Blue 1, Blue 2, Green 3, Orange B, and Red 3, are used heavily in various candies, breakfast cereals and even yoghurt.
7. **Irradiation to kill dangerous organisms** in beef, pork, chicken, lamb, herbs, spices, flour, fruits and vegetables. The European Union (EU) only allows it on dried spices, herbs and vegetable based seasonings.
8. **Bleached flour** used in all white bread and some wheat bread.
9. **Partially hydrogenated oils** are completely banned or severely restricted in some EU countries.
10. **Many chemicals such as aspartame and saccharine and preservatives like titanium dioxide** used in sugar substitutes and to make food white and bright such as in toothpaste. **(6)**

.
This chapter ends with a phrase from my other book: "The common philosophy of the United States on this subject seems to be that a food or chemical is innocent or harmless until proven guilty or harmful. European philosophy on the same matter has it opposite; a product is considered harmful or guilty until proven harmless or innocent."

Wellness in a Toxic World

2 Lab Tests

In alternative preventive medicine, many lab tests are ordered for a multitude of health issues. After twenty seven years of clinical experience I have migrated to the camp advocating fewer tests ordered to attain as well as maintain the highest degree of health.

I usually order a CMP (complete metabolic panel), lipid panel, complete thyroid panel, and when deemed necessary a CBC (complete blood count) with auto differential. I may do some heavy metal toxicity analysis using both hair and urine and several hormone panel tests if problems are not improving. I also use genetic testing which provides extremely valuable information which can change someone's life after other treatments have been unsuccessful. A lot of the training I have had includes using functional analysis which can identify problems before they arise as overt symptoms. This analysis lowers the threshold of conventional "pathological " lab values. As Datis Kharrazian DC states, "the problem with conventional blood range values is they often fail to discover an underlying precipitating problem until it is well established."**(7)** An example of this problem is obvious in the test for blood glucose levels. Conventional labs have the normal range at 65 or 70 -100mg/dL.; normal values for blood glucose levels should between 85-100 mg/dL. There is too much of a range with the conventional levels for the blood sugar to be stable. When blood sugar crashes, a person will eat more food in an attempt to bring up the sugar level, but he will then need more insulin to carry this increased sugar into the cells. If someone continuously goes on this up and down sugar merry go round, insulin output levels will have to continually increase to account for the cells' decrease in insulin sensitivity that results. Sooner or later, the pancreas will not be able to keep up with the demand for the high amounts of sugar eaten and insufficient insulin will be produced, resulting in type two diabetes. Eventually the pancreas may lose the ability to produce any insulin and the patient is then diagnosed with type one diabetes. If a blood glucose level is 70 one day and then the next it is 90 in a recurrent pattern, there may be a problem starting even though the "conventional" ranges are maintained. These ranges are set up with a wait and see philosophy instead of the preventative cautious approach functional medicine uses. Thus, for conventional medicine, below 85 is hypoglycemic and 100-126 (insulin resistant in which the receptor sites are resistant to insulin) is pre-diabetic: 127 or above is diabetes. I must discuss the conventional ranges versus the functional ranges using logical reasoning so you can make up your own mind which values are more accurate.

Hem AIC (hemoglobin) conventional values should be less than 7% of total hemoglobin while functional ranges less than 4.1-5.7%. The Hem AIC measures the amount of glucose which combines with hemoglobin in the blood. Normal red blood cells have a lifespan of 120 days, and the higher the glucose in the blood, the more it will combine with hemoglobin; this process is irreversible. This test will measure the average amount of glucose combining with hemoglobin or glycation, on a sub type of hemoglobin or A1C and the average levels of blood glucose for a 2-3 month period before the test. Those people with levels above 5.7% indicate poor management of long term blood glucose and are possibly in the insulin resistant state known as pre-diabetes. "Research indicates that most patients will progress through various stages of insulin resistance and glucose intolerance before becoming a classic diabetic." The stages include: normal glucose tolerance followed by hypoglycemia (often due to hyperinsulinemia) then insulin insensitivity/resistance followed eventually by type two diabetes. **(8)** The flip side of a high AIC is a low AIC. As stated above, lower blood sugar, or hypoglycemia is the precursor to diabetes; the levels of glucose less than 80 and an AIC of less than 4.45 cannot be to be maintained in the blood. We must keep in mind that lower levels of glucose and AIC can be just as dangerous as higher levels.

Cholesterol, as I mentioned previously, is one of the most controversial items tested. The conventional ranges are 125-200 mg/dL, functional ranges between 150-220 mg/dL. Cholesterol has been blamed as a causal factor of heart disease for too long. Finally, some in the medical profession are starting to agree that cholesterol was unjustly implicated as a major risk for strokes and heart attacks. I discussed at length in my other book that cardiovascular surgeon Dwight Lundell MD told the public to wake up and stop eating the low fat/ low cholesterol diet. According to him, by following these conventional dietary recommendations, the public is doing more harm than good resulting in increasing record numbers of heart disease-related deaths. Presently, there is still no definitive proof of a cholesterol - heart disease link. Moreover, those dying of heart attacks generally have had the lowest total cholesterol levels. The well known Framingham Study of 1948 involving 6.000 people compared those who ate large amount of saturated fats and cholesterol with those who ate much less. In 2013 the director reiterated the incredible conclusion that, "the more saturated fat one ate, the more cholesterol one ate, the more calories one ate, the lower the person's serum cholesterol. We found that the people who ate the most cholesterol, ate the most saturated fat, and ate the most calories, weighed the least and were the most physically active." The Framingham study did show an increased risk of cardiovascular disease for those who weighed more, but there was an inverse correlation between weight gain and cholesterol with fat and cholesterol dietary intake. I recommend the book *The Great Cholesterol Con* by Anthony Colpo MD for those who want to investigate this subject more thoroughly. Let me summarize the importance of cholesterol to the human body. Found in every cell, an essential component of the cellular membrane, cholesterol is crucial for membrane fluidity and determining what enters and exits the cell. Importantly, it is a free radical scavenger and protects the body from free radical damage. Cholesterol is the raw material for the body's hormones. If your cholesterol is high, the liver filtration system is clogged with toxic materials resulting in abnormal hormone levels. **(9)** Furthermore, one half of the brain's dry weight is composed of cholesterol.; a critical substances the body requires to survive!

LDLs, low density lipoproteins and HDLs, high density lipoproteins are two forms of cholesterol. LDLs carry the cholesterol and most of the essential fatty acids from the liver to the tissues of the body. Functional values should be less than 120 mg/dL, conventional ranges for LDLs 60-130 mg/dL. HDLs are the lipoproteins which transport cholesterol from the peripheral tissues and blood vessel walls to the liver where they can be turned in bile salts. Functional values should be greater than 55 mg/dL and conventional values between 40-90 mg/dL. These two have an inverse relationship, as one increases the other decreases. Since the LDLs bring the cholesterol from the liver to the tissues it is labeled "bad cholesterol" increasing the chances of atherosclerosis while HDLs are thought to be "good cholesterol" because they bring the cholesterol from these tissues to the liver therefore protecting against arteriosclerosis. When higher levels of LDLs and lower HDLs are present, there is an increased risk of coronary artery disease, diabetes and syndrome X which is indicative of high blood pressure, glucose intolerance and high triglycerides or fats.

Triglycerides, or fats in the blood, are from two sources: diet and liver. The conventional values are 30-150 mg/dL and functional values should be between 75-100 mg/dL. If a body metabolizes fats and carbohydrates properly, the triglyceride value should be about one half of the total cholesterol value. Dick Weatherby N.D. and Scott Fergusson describe diet and triglycerides succinctly; I will quote and summarize a paragraph from their book, *Blood Chemistry and CBC Analysis*. Two main facts to remember about triglycerides and diet are: "Elevated or decreased triglycerides alone are almost never the problem and elevated dietary fat is almost never the sole cause of elevated serum triglycerides." Yes, you guessed it- it is those infamous sugary carbohydrates leading to blood sugar dysfunction reflecting a breakdown in the body's regulatory capacity. Thus a diet high in carbohydrates and junk hydrogenated oils may contribute to elevated triglycerides.**(10)**

Another component of the lab test is for Iron. Conventional values are 30-170 ug/dL and functional ones, 85-130 ug/dL. Most iron in the body is in the form of hemoglobin; the remaining is stored in the spleen, liver and bone marrow. Because iron is such a crucial element of overall health, I must stress that simply testing only for the level of iron in the blood (serum iron) does not provide enough significant clinical information, serum ferritin and TIBC (total iron biding capacity) should also be ordered to totally access whether or not anemia is present and to what degree. The main storage form of iron in the body is called ferritin. The body tries to keep serum iron levels steady so the storage form, or ferritin, will then be the most sensitive to detect iron deficiency on a blood test. Normal conventional ferritin ranges are between 10-232 ng/mL, functional values 10-132ng/mL for females and 33-262 ng/mL for males. TIBC conventional ranges are 250-350 ug/dL which also happens to be identical to the functional values! With levels too high, there is a hereditary condition in which the body absorbs too much iron that is deposited in the tissues especially the liver; this can lead to cardiovascular, liver problems, dementia and arteriosclerosis to name a few. Dietary sources include iron tablets, pots and pans and some drinking water. TIBC measures the amount of iron in the blood carried by the protein transferrin. A decreased serum iron, ferritin, and TIBC along with some other RBC indices is highly suggestive of iron deficiency anemia; these tests assess anemia and monitor an iron overload.

Uric acid conventional values are 2.2-7.7mg/dL , functional values 3.5-5.9

mg/dL for males and 3.0-5.5 mg/mg/dL for females. These levels indicate the end product of protein utilization in the liver. High levels usually indicate gout in which the uric acid crystals deposit in the tissues, especially the tophi or big toe in men and the ankle and knee in females. Keep in mind however, that an over production of uric acid also occurs in other health problems causing excessive tissue destruction and inflammation. Dietary sources of purines from dark meats and high protein foods are usually implicated in this and should be avoided when levels are high; but chemical and physical stressors are the most common reason for increased levels. One major source is oxidative stress, heart disease and high triglycerides. In fact over ¾ of high triglyceride cardiac patients will present with elevated uric acid levels. **(11)** Moreover, we must also consider the body's ability to normally excrete uric acid; the levels will rise with excretory problems. The kidneys excrete 66% or so and the remaining third goes out with the stool. By testing uric acid levels, kidney function is also evaluated. As a marker for oxidative stress and a screening for heart disease, evaluating any suspect inflammatory/circulation problem, are the reasons for running this test.

For RBC (red blood cells) conventional ranges are 4.6-6.0 x10 12th/L in males and 3.8-5.1 in females. The optimal, functional range is from 4.2-4.9x10$9^{th}$/L and 4.0-4.5 respectively. These cells simultaneously carry oxygen from the lungs to the body while transferring carbon dioxide from the tissues to the lungs. The RBC test measures the amount of red blood cells or erythrocytes found in one cubic millimeter of blood. Suspecting anemia and dehydration are the two reasons to run this test which also aids in evaluating the liver's ability to cleanse the blood.

For Hemoglobin conventional values are 12.5-17.0 g/dL for males and 11.5-15.0 g/dL for females. Functional ranges are 14.0-15.0 g/dL and 13.5-14.5g/dL respectively. Hemoglobin is the major molecule in the blood which functions to transport oxygen to the cells. Other tests include MCV (Mean corpuscular volume), MCH (mean corpuscular hemoglobin) and MCHC (Mean corpuscular hemoglobin concentration). Conventional values for MCV 80-90 fL and functional values 82-89.9 fL. MCH conventional values 27-34 pg and functional values are 28-31.9 pg. Conventional values for MCHC are 32-36 g/dL and functional values are 32-35g/dL. HCT(hematocrit) refers to the percentage of the cell volume the packed red blood cells take up. Conventional values are 36%-50% for males and 34%-44% for females. Functional/optimal ranges are 40% - 48% and 37% - 44% respectfully. RDW (red cell distribution width) indicates the amount of abnormal size variation of red blood cells. For the most part, variations of all of these blood indices test values are concerned with various form of anemias. (I realize the reader may skim over some of the technical information here).

When the hemoglobin is extracted from the red blood cells, bilirubin forms and must be transported back to the liver to become water soluble so that it can be excreted with the bile in the feces. Both conventional and functional values for total bilirubin are the same at 0.1-1.2 mg/dl. Total bilirubin consists of two forms, direct and indirect.. The conventional values for unconjugated direct bilirubin are 0.0.2 mg/dL and indirect conjugated bilirubin values are 0.1-1.0 mg/dL. The former is bilirubin that is not conjugated or made water soluble yet, and if increased it indicates a liver or gallbladder problem. When indirect bilirubin has been conjugated to water soluble, and if increased, this usually means the red blood cells are being destroyed. It is important to analyze both forms of indirect and direct forms on a blood chemistry; otherwise, the total bilirubin has much less clinical significance. **(12)**

Platelet count conventional ranges are 155 - 385 x 10^{9th}/L and 155 x 10^{3rd}/mm 3rd are the functional or optimal ranges. This test monitors bleeding disorders since the platelets are the smallest formed elements in the blood and necessary for clotting. Hardening of the arteries or plaque buildup can cause the count to be high, and many things such as infection, heavy metals toxicity, oxidative stress and DRUG REACTIONS can cause the numbers to drop below normal. Some drugs known to drop your platelet count are the Sulfas and Quinidine.

WBC (white blood cells) also known as leukocytes, are divided into two groups granulocytes and agranulocytes. Within the first group we have neutrophils, basophils and eosinophils. The second group consists of monocytes and lymphocytes. The conventional ranges are 3.7-11 x 10^{9th}/L and functional ranges are 5.0-.75 x 10^{9th}/L. Acute or recent infection is associated with an elevated WBC, whereas a chronic or long term infection results in a lower WBC count. Gastrointestinal distress is evaluated by looking at the monocytes and eosinophil values. If both are elevated the probability of parasitic infection is high. The test is mainly run to assess the immune system's ability to fight infection and inflammation and to evaluate whether or not an infection is present.

The thyroid panel of tests warrants a repetition of information I covered in my previous book. Millions of hypothyroid and Hashimotos sufferers in America remain undiagnosed because their blood test results do not fall into the "conventional" blood ranges established by the medical community. In order to fully evaluate thyroid function, several essential tests must be ordered. The TSH (thyroid stimulating hormone) is the most commonly used test to evaluate the thyroid gland. The hypothalamic-anterior pituitary-thyroid negative feedback system secretes a Thyroid releasing hormone which then causes the anterior pituitary to secret TSH. This stimulates the thyroid to secrete T-4 and T-3, two hormones which then act negatively to suppress TSH controlling its production. The TSH is the most sensitive test for primary hypothyroidism and to evaluate the thyroid. However, if a clinical symptomatic picture is present, and the TSH is normal, then other tests must be run to rule out problems with the pituitary or hypothalamus glands. Conventional ranges for TSH are anywhere from .35-5.5 mlU/L. Functional ranges are not totally agreed upon. The values I use are between 1.8-3.0 mlU/L ; others go by a 2.0-4.4mlU/L range. If TSH levels are below normal it is a low functioning thyroid or hypothyroid and if above the normal range, the thyroid is hyperthyroid. Think of it this way: a high level of T3 indicates that it must have been a high level of TSH secreted to stimulate it and since it is still not "used up" and measurable, no more TSH is needed by the body. The opposite is then true. If there are low levels of T-3 and T-4 in the blood, more TSH must be secreted to stimulate more. In T-3, the most active form of thyroid hormone, conventional ranges are 80-230ng/dL. Functional ranges are between 100-230ng/dL. If high this indicates hyperthyroidism or could possibly mean iodine deficiency; if low this could indicate primary hypothyroidism. T4 conventional ranges are 4.8-13.2 mcg/dL., functional ranges are 6.0-12.0 mcg/dL. T4 is the major hormone secreted by the thyroid gland and must to be converted to the active form T3 in order to be utilized. 60% of it is converted in the liver, 20% converted in the gut (if the right bacterial flora are present), and the rest in other body tissues. When evaluating the thyroid gland some doctors only order TT3 (total t3) and TT4 (total t4). Because, each are largely attached to protein molecules and not ready for metabolic processes, tests for FT4 (free T4) and FT3 (free T3) are necessary; unbound and more open to tissue receptors, they therefore paint a more accurate picture of thyroid function. **(13)** T3 uptake is another part of the thyroid panel which measures changes in the number of thyroid binding proteins, and is useful evaluating an increase in T4 by ruling out any lab error. Conventional values are 22-39% of uptake. Functional values are 27-39% of uptake. (There are different classifications of hypothyroid but it is complicated). The most common thyroid condition is thyroiditis or inflammation of the thyroid. 90% of those suffering from this have been found to have Hashimoto's Autoimmune Thyroiditis, a combination of hypo and hyperthyroidism in which symptoms seem to alternate between the two conditions. Two other tests can be ordered to confirm the autoimmune thyroiditis or Hashimotos. TPO (thyroid peroxidase) antibodies and TGB (thyroxine globulin binding) antibodies are both indicators of an autoimmune thyroid. The conventional values are anything less than 35 IU/mL for the former and less than 20 IU/mL latter. One must remember however, that if a patient has blood drawn during a period when they are mostly symptom free, there may not be a higher count of these antibodies and an abnormal condition may go undetected. Triggers such as gluten and an active infection, however, will usually send these antibody readings through the roof.

The CRP (c-reactive protein) test measures rapid non- specific increases in inflammation; it is an inflammatory marker. It also can be used to monitor the effects of supplements or medication in lowering systemic/whole body inflammation. The HsCRP (high sensitivity) test is a good indicator of cardiovascular risk. Many functional medicine practitioners maintain that the best functional value is 0-3mg/L. On the contrary, many conventional lab results run the Cardio CRP breaking down the values as follows: less than 1 is a lower cardiovascular risk,. 1-3.0 is average cardiovascular risk, 3.1-10 is higher relative cardiovascular risk. Greater than 10.0 may be associated with infection and inflammation if persistently elevated after retesting. This test is found to be a more sensitive one than the SED (sedimentation) rate in identifying inflammation in the body. (The sedimentation rate is run to look for tissue destruction and inflammation.)

Homocysteine is another inflammatory marker to be made from another amino acid called methionine. Some dietary sources of methionine are fish, eggs, and certain nuts. Normally, homocysteine gets converted in the body to SAMe (S-Adenosyl methionine) and glutathione which have great health benefits such as arthritis prevention to anti-oxidant protection. B vitamins and Zinc are the two main ingredients needed for this conversion; a deficiency of either of these two substances results in a build-up of homocysteine levels. This is a good indicator of digestive dysfunction. For example, parasites are known to devour B vitamins. Furthermore, hydrochloric acid (stomach acid) is also needed for homocysteine metabolism or breakdown. This breakdown of homocysteine is also the key for the neurotransmitter synthesis of acetylcholine needed for memory and for myelin production needed for nerve conduction. Conventional values are between 5.4- 11.9 umol/L while the functional should be tighter at 7.0- 9.0 umol/L. The mineral sodium, comprising 90% of the body's extracellular fluid, has conventional values of 135-146 mmol/L and functional values of 135-140 mmol/L. The adrenal glands, particularly the adrenal cortex with its steroid hormone aldosterone, regulates the body's sodium balance by holding or decreasing it's excretion in the urine. Thus this test evaluates adrenal gland health. (The sodium blood test is not as sensitive to altered levels compared to the urine test). Sodium also maintains the acid base balance of the blood and the urine and has an intricate relationship with potassium, another mineral. Together they form the sodium potassium pump which enables their transport across cell membranes. This pump is intricately related to other mineral electrolytes in your blood and other body fluids that carry an electric charge. Conventional values for potassium are 3.5-5.3 mmol/L and the functional optimal ranges are 4.0-4.5 mmol/L. Like sodium, potassium is also a measure of adrenal health and the acid/base balance of the body. A negatively charged 90% intracellular ion, potassium is the opposing balance to the positively 90% extracellular charged ion sodium.. The adrenal hormone aldosterone causes excretion of potassium to balance its lack of excreted sodium. Chloride, another important electrolyte is also mostly extracellular and hangs out with sodium in the form of sodium chloride and, for the most part, acts with sodium. The conventional values of chloride are 97- 107 mmol/L with the optimal ranges being 100-106 mmol./L. This test is one of the markers for hypochlorohydria or lower stomach acid and is also involved with acid base balance of the body tissues. **In my previous book, I described in detail, the difference between body pH and stomach pH and the huge role they play in total body health.** Carbon Dioxide refers to the amount alkaline or base bound as bicarbonate in the blood. This bicarbonate carbon dioxide's job is to neutralize or balance lactic and hydrochloric acid. The conventional values are 23-32mmol/L with optimal functional ranges set at 25-30mmol/L. Although this test is run to assess tissue pH, keep in mind that chloride, blood gases, and anion gap-which I will discuss next, are needed for full carbon dioxide evaluation. (Carbon dioxide not in the form of bicarbonate is a dissolved acid and is regulated by the lungs). Anion gap refers to the different amounts of the serum cations or positively charged ions and the serum anions or negatively charged ions. Thus, we are talking about the difference between the amount of sodium/potassium and the amount of Carbon dioxide/bicarbonate and chloride. Conventional values are 6-16 mmol/L, functional values are 7-12 mmol/L. This test, like the electrolyte test rationale immediately preceding it, measures body tissue pH. Calcium is the next test. The conventional values for calcium are 9.5-10.8 mg/dL and functional ranges are 9.2-10.1 mg/dL. Most people believe that they are deficient in calcium from dietary sources, however; research has found that it is the inability to absorb calcium due to: the lack of stomach acid, a deficiency in magnesium, phosphorous, B vitamins and/or fats. Calcium must be absorbed in the upper part of the small intestine. However, if there is a decrease in hydrochloric acid, this means undigested food will be dumped into the small intestine and putrify. Most calcium in the blood plasma is in the ionized form regulated by the parathyroid and Vit D. Thus the calcium test is ordered to ascertain digestive function and parathyroid function. Magnesium, the next mineral with a conventional

range of 1.5-2.3mg/dL and functional range of greater than 2 mg/dL and is intricately related to calcium as potassium is to sodium; therefore you cannot effect one without the other. Most people are aware of the indicators of magnesium deficiency including cardiac arrhythmias and leg cramps but may not heard of chocolate cravings and chronic constipation.
For phosphorous, the conventional ranges are 2.5-4.5 mg/dL and functional ranges 3.0-4.0 mg/dL. This mineral, like calcium, with whom it shares an inverse relationship, is also regulated by the parathyroid. When evaluating serum phosphorous calcium must be assessed to get a complete picture. Indicators for ordering are the same as with calcium: to evaluate the parathyroid and digestive function. Creatinine has conventional values of .5-1.05 mg/dL. and functional ranges .7-1.1 mg/dL and is tested to evaluate kidney function. Creatinine is the waste product of creatine, an amino acid in the muscles of vertebrates essential for muscle contraction. When it is broken down it can be measured in the blood. In general, those with more muscle mass have higher amounts of creatinine than those with a decreased amount. Consequently, it is not as sensitive as BUN, our next test in detecting early kidney disease. BUN (Blood Urea Nitrogen) is a measure of the difference between the production and clearance of urea the chief end product of protein digestion. This is made almost entirely in the liver and removed almost entirely by the kidneys. Conventional ranges are 7-25 mg/dL and functional ranges 6-22 mg/dL. This is a more sensitive test to detect kidney disease than creatinine because its serum values rise quicker in early stage kidney disease. Alkaline phosphatase is the next blood test. Conventional values are 25-120 U/L and functional values 70-100 U/L. This is an isoenzyme from the metaloprotein family of enzymes and is zinc dependent; decreased alkaline phosphatase levels have been associated with a zinc deficiency. This isoenzyme originates in the bone, intestines, liver, kidney and placenta. The test evaluates liver or gallbladder dysfunction, monitors bone disorders and as a tumor marker. Many times elevation of this isoenzyme is also associated with drug induced liver damage. AST (aspartate amino transferase) is next, an enzyme located in muscle, liver, heart, kidney, and lungs. When there is tissue destruction in one of these areas this enzyme goes into the blood. Conventional values are 0-40 U/L and functional values 10-30 U/L. AST is more specific for cardiac problems and can also be indicative of a B6 deficiency. ALT (alanine aminotransferase) is the next test. This enzyme, like AST, is prevalent in skeletal muscle, heart and kidney tissues. However, this is most prevalent in the liver and much less in the other tissues. The conventional values for this enzyme are 0-45 U/L and the functional values are 10-30 U/L. This is very similar functionally to AST; however, it is more specific to liver and gallbladder problems and less to cardiac. GGTP is another test evaluating an enzyme that is very prevalent in liver tissue, and also present in smaller

amounts in the kidney, prostate and pancreas. The conventional values are 1-70 U/L and functional values are 10-30 U/L. This test is very sensitive to liver problems and biliary obstruction; in fact it is more sensitive than both the Alkaline phosphatase and ALT enzymes for evaluating liver dysfunction; it is also run to monitor alcoholism. In the next test, LDH (lactate dehydrogenase) indicates certain enzymes involvement in carbohydrate metabolism. Conventional values are 1-240 U/L and functional values are 140-200 U/L. Like the previously aforementioned enzymes, LDH is found in many body tissues and especially the heart, liver, and kidney, skeletal muscle, red blood cells, and lungs. This test is run to look for tissue damage associated with those areas.

I tried to paint a symptomatic picture for the rationale for ordering the preceding last five enzymes which evaluate the liver, gallbladder and bile duct/pancreas. Countless Americans have gallstones; in fact, according to health professional Andreas Moritz, author of *The Amazing Liver and Gallbladder Flush*, most people have congestion of bile and suffer from gallstones. For those of you who have had your gallbladder removed, do not feel left out he says; most people have gallstones in their hepatic ducts located in the liver. **Thus if someone is having pain between the shoulder blades which does not seem to be mechanical/ related to motion, or if one becomes easily intoxicated from alcohol, or is sensitive to perfumes or chemical smells, has a headache over one eye, or suffers from hemorrhoids, he could have some biliary obstruction or gall stones**. Over the past twenty-five years I have had countless patients who exemplified aspects of the symptomatic picture I just painted. They had gone to their family physician only to end up with gallbladder removal surgery. I urge those with any known confirmed medical gallbladder problems to read Moritz's book before taking any action. It's very fascinating the way the author explains how backed up bile and toxins which form gallstones can then influence every other body system and be the cause or start of many future disease processes. Albumin, one the major blood proteins produced primarily in the liver and is the major transport of many substances such as drugs and hormones, is the next blood test considered. Osmotic pressure between blood vessels and tissue fluids is due to albumin. Conventional values are 3.5-5.5 g/dL. and functional values are 4.0-5.0 g/dL. This test assesses digestive function and hydration.

Globulin levels refers to proteins produced in the liver, (see how important the liver is with all of these lab tests?) reticuloendothelial system (lymphatic capillaries and connective tissues) and other body tissues which also transport substances in the blood. The globulins make up the antibody system and clotting proteins. Conventional values are 2.0-3.9 g/dL and functional values 2.4-2.8 g/dL. This test evaluates digestive function and inflammatory or immune problems. For the Albumin/Globulin ratio test, conventional values are 1.1-2.5 and functional values are 1.5-2.0. High or low ratios indicate liver and immune dysfunction. There is also a test for total serum protein which is a combination of albumin and total globulin. Conventional values are 6.0-8.5 g/dL and functional values are 6.9-7.4 g/dL. Many factors affect protein absorption such as a lack of stomach acid (HCL). Dysfunction of the pancreas and small intestine can also affect this absorption. Thus indicators for the total protein test are to assess nutritional deficiencies, dehydration and digestive dysfunction. Keep in mind that the total protein level can be in the normal range but the total globulin or albumin can be increased or decreased individually; that is why you must assess globin and albumin levels individually as well. The last item on a blood chemistry that is routinely tested is Vitamin D, a fat soluble vitamin which is really a prohormone, biologically inactive that must be converted to its active forms. There are two forms of Vitamin D, the storage form also known as 25 (OH) with a conventional value of 10-55 ng/mL and functional values 35-80ng/mL. The active form known as Vit D 1,25 has conventional values of 24-65pg/mL and functional levels of up to 75pg/mL. The inactive 25 (OH) requires sufficient magnesium to be converted to the active form in the kidneys. If a doctor only tests for the inactive form, the patient will not know how the body is able to convert this to the biologically active form. A situation can arise in which the active form 1,25 is too high and suppress thyroid and cortisol receptors adversely affecting the thyroid and blood sugar values. **Vit D deficiency plays a HUGE role in immunity and as an anti-inflammatory agent. Interestingly, Vitamin D is essential for apoptosis or normal cell death. This does not occur in cancer patients whose cells are multiplying out of control. The precursor to Vitamin D, since it is really a hormone, is cholesterol. How do the statin drug that many Americans are taking, figure in all of this? One could infer that cholesterol lowering medications may increase cancer rates?**

There you have it. That is the blood work I order most often on patients. I also do heavy metal testing using both hair and urine analysis. On a personal note, I had a hair analysis done when I was twenty nine years old and still have the results booklet from the same company I use today called Analytical Research Labs; I trust their findings. Many of the naysayers over the years, arguing that hair analysis is bogus or inaccurate are mainly from those in conventional medicine. Blood and urine analyses obviously are the standards for evaluating body fluids but fail to take into account the biochemical processes that occur inside of the cells. Since it is not feasible to perform a whole body biopsy to evaluate the cells, other cells such as hair, readily available can be used. Extensive research has shown that the hair cells and cells of other body tissues are equally as valid with their level of mineral when tested; they reach the same conclusion. Minerals are extremely important to sustain life because they control the body's enzymes and hormones.

Hair analysis is able to reveal minerals stored for the past three months or so. Not only a test for mineral evaluation but it is also a biochemical picture of one's immune function, metabolism, carbohydrate sensitivity, glandular function and more. Eventually, a mineral imbalance will show up in the blood but unfortunately not usually until a person has overt symptoms. A hair analysis screening can find an imbalance before it becomes chronic or severe; thus it supplies one more tool to add to the proverbial toolbox, by providing more indicators and removing guesswork when recommending what types of diet and nutritional supplements or oils one should take.

ARLs (analytical research labs) uses ideal standards when they test hair and not just the average results of past specimens as most other hair analysis companies do. Their main nutrient mineral levels test is with the following minerals: calcium, magnesium, sodium, potassium, iron, copper, manganese, zinc, chromium, selenium, and phosphorous. Additional minerals tested for include: nickel, cobalt, molybdenum, lithium and boron. Their toxic metal analysis involves: lead, mercury, cadmium, arsenic and aluminum. There are no conventional values for hair analysis because the medical establishment does not consider it a valid method of testing. The values given, therefore, are functional. For example, a calcium/potassium ratio should be 4:1 known as "the thyroid ratio" because these minerals regulate thyroid activity. The adrenal glands are inextricably linked to the thyroid via the HPA (hypothalamic pituitary adrenal) axis. For proper function, there needs to be a calcium/potassium ratio of 4:1 and a sodium/potassium ratio of 2.5:1.

When giving nutritional advice first, this company also recognizes individual body chemistry by categorizing each patient as a slow, medium or fast oxidizer, thus avoiding mismatching nutrients leading to detrimental health effects. The "oxidation rate" is determined by how long it takes the body to convert food to energy.

Let me offer a scenario of the ramifications of a copper and zinc imbalance. A higher protein diet is known to increase the secretion of thyroxin, a thyroid hormone, and the efficiency of food oxidation or burning. A complication of this is that different kinds of proteins contains copper in different amounts. For example, vegetarian proteins such as soybeans, tofu, avocado, nuts and grains are high in copper thus the adrenal glands are compromised; they cannot stimulate synthesis of cerculoplasmin, the main copper binding protein made in the liver, and the copper therefore gets deposited in various tissues throughout the body rather than excreted with the bile. The result is a copper toxicity. **(14)** I was astonished to find that out of all of the hair analysis ARL conducts, 70-80% of the specimens show an adrenal insufficiency! It is therefore logical to assume only that copper toxicity is one of the most common imbalances they find; especially considering the super- sized portion of protein in restaurant food. Keep in mind that zinc and copper are inversely proportional. Of the various types of proteins greatly consumed, red meat is one of the highest in zinc. Yet the copper toxic patient loses their taste for red meat due to their zinc deficiency. In an afflicted patient, until the adrenal glands insufficiency is corrected, fish, eggs, and chicken protein should be eaten with digestive enzymes and HCL (hydrochloric acid) to ensure proper digestion. (I will expand on digestive enzymes and HCL later).

Heavy metal analysis can also be performed by testing urine. A detoxification agent is used prior to the test to ensure an objective method of evaluating the accumulation of toxic metals. A chronic long term accumulation of toxic metals, not the acute poisoning which is very rare, can have devastating adverse health effects leading to a multitude of chronic illnesses. Many doctors test essential elements with the toxic metal analysis, using a detoxification agent, because many toxic metals will take essential minerals with them when excreted from the body.

Genetic testing, a cutting edge diagnostic tool, is another method I have begun to use. Dr. John Thomas, an expert in this field and colleague of mine, has provided much of the important critical information that I use. Therefore I must summarize some important points from his latest methylation webinar on our forum. He explains that genetic testing provides more sophisticated explanations needed for a patient not responding to all of the therapies he has received so far. What this test reports is SNPs or single nucleotide polymorphisms which constitute genetic abnormalities, both major and minor ones. Obviously we will focus on the major- life changing ones and disregard the less insignificant ones. His
report explains such categories as allergies, clotting factors, detoxification, immune system (IGG- IGA- IGE), mitochondria, thyroid, and the methylation process. The categories are then color coded as green, yellow and red with green being good, yellow being not so good and red being really bad. We have two copies of the majority of our genes from birth-

one from each parent. This report addresses SNPs from a person's unique DNA sequence to see if one or both copies of the gene has a mutation at a specific location on a specific gene. The SNPs are variants which naturally occur on genes altering their functions. This could determine hair, eye or skin color for example. Other SNPs have functional effects on genes giving us insight on how well key body functions are performed which then determines level of health. There are heterozygous and homozygous terms used by geneticists to denote whether one or both copies of a gene are mutated. Someone with a heterozygous mutation for instance, has one fully functioning copy of a gene besides the one that is mutated. A homozygous mutation, however, has both copies of a mutated gene. It is important to realize that this is not an indication of a defective or non- functioning gene; it simply means the gene function is working with an "altered" level of efficiency. This could sometimes mean a decreased or an increased level. It may also mean that the regulatory mechanism, which is normally a part of the gene's expression, is absent. Most often these mutations have been with us since birth, and we will have them throughout our lives. These are inherited mutations and have been passed down from previous generations of parents and grandparents and may continue to be passed on to future generations. This may provide an answer to why certain conditions seem to "run in the family" and this is also where the phrase "I inherited this height from my dad" comes from.

This leads us to the topic of epigenetics or how our genes are influenced by the environment. **Although it is a fact that we cannot change our genetic code, research has revealed that our gene expression is not only determined by heredity factors but can indeed be influenced by environmental stressors, diet, and toxic load.** Furthermore, certain genes can be over or under expressed with some disease processes.
This means if we can learn more about how genes are regulated, not only can we optimize their genetic expression but overall health as well. **WOW!**

Correlating the genetic findings with the patient's symptomatology allows a doctor to make treatment recommendations accordingly. Therefore, I only review select genes within someone's complete genetic profile. Remember, because you have gene mutations or alterations does not mean there will be problems with the functioning of that gene or that there is a present disease or pathology. **Research does indicate, however, that certain gene mutations may cause specific problems in certain individuals**.
There are many categories to consider but I focus only on the most important ones for that particular patient's condition.

One category I select is <u>Methylation</u> because of it's importance and relationship to so many prevalent chronic diseases. Methyl groups (CH3) are needed to prevent "mutated" genes from being expressed. They get depleted from the SAD (white sugar, salt, and flour), junk polyunsaturated oils, EMFs from cell phones and towers, dirty electricity, pesticides, herbicides, high fructose corn syrup, other genetically modified foods and a lot of emotional stress. (Methyl groups are created from adequate amount of hydrochloric acid (stomach acid); however, a problem arises after age thirty when the body continues to produces less). Methyl groups are essential for: DNA/RNA synthesis which determines turning off and on genes, neurotransmitter production such as dopamine and serotonin, the breakdown of estrogen and testosterone, immune cell creation, protective myelin sheath on nerves, detoxification of chemicals and toxins, and energy production. With insufficient methylation, the body it is more susceptible to such chronic diseases as cancer, diabetes, thyroid disorders, neurological disorders like Parkinson's, Alzheimer's, dementia, hormonal disorders like ovarian cysts, fibroids with PMS, fibromyalgia, chronic fatigue syndrome, autoimmune disorders, ADHD, insomnia, anxiety, Lyme disease, gut issues, heart disease etc. I will briefly mention a few genes in the methylation category and how their mutations correlate with patient symptoms.

The first is the MTHFR C677T gene mutation, one of the key MTHFR (methyl tetrahydrofolate reductase) enzyme SNPs. This indicates that the enzyme may have trouble performing its normal functions resulting in high levels of homocysteine- remember this from the blood test
discussion just previously. High homocysteine can be a factor in the onset of bi-polar disorder, peripheral neuropathy, Multiple Sclerosis and Alzheimer's disease, to name a few. If heterozygous (from one parent) it indicates a 30% reduction of normal methylation function. Homozygous (from both parents) indicates a 70% reduction in MTHF production. My wife Becky's genetic screening revealed a heterozygous SNP with this gene, meaning a 30% reduction in cell methylation function. The impairment of this enzyme can cause or contribute to chemical sensitivity, blood clots and stroke, to name just a few. Ever since I have known Becky, she hardly ever bled when accidently cutting herself. As a matter of fact, I would often remark that her blood was like sludge. Since she starting using do-TERRA essential oils and supplements, I noticed that she has normal blood flow after a cut. She is also sensitive to many chemicals and perfume/colognes and almost develops an immediate headache after inhaling a whiff of either. Remember, as I stated earlier, this headache is indicative of gallstones for which I recommend a flush.

The other key MTHFR gene SNP is A 1298C. Unlike the first one, this does not lead to higher levels of homocysteine, but instead can affect neurotransmitter function. Produced in the brain, neurotransmitters are chemicals such as serotonin and dopamine which control our mood and smooth movement. This mutation is associated with depression, anxiety, migraines, dementia, schizophrenia, and Parkinson's. The normal 1298C plays an important role in mood regulation and addictive behavior. A heterozygous A1298C gene mutation- from one parent, is indicative of a 10% reduction in MTHF production whereas a homozygous gene mutation- from both parents, indicates a 30% reduction of MTHF. There is also a mixed 677/1298 compound heterozygous gene SNP indicative of a 40-50% reduction in MTHF production. I have the heterozygous SNP for this gene meaning a 10% reduction in methylation function. Luckily, I do not have any of the symptoms associated with neurotransmitter function but it is something to always watch out for.

There are many other important SNPs in this methylation category that I correlate with a patient's symptoms. For example, someone may have insomnia. After trying a lot of various remedies with only mild success, I find a mutated GAD gene. This results in a decrease in the body's ability to convert glutamic acid into GABA, a neurotransmitter which stabilizes the brain by preventing an overexcited state resulting in a calming effect. The patient with inadequate amounts of GABA will exhibit a dissatisfaction with life, spasticity, low muscle tone, and sleeping problems. This patient will need more nutritional support to specifically increase or restore GABA production. Without the genetic test, we would have only given sleep support not knowing underlying reason for the sleeplessness. Becky has a heterozygous SNPs for the GAD gene and suffers from sleep disturbances mostly due to, she claims, "her mind going 100 miles per hour." With supplements, oils and diet, her sleeping difficulty occurs less often; however, when she strays from her diet or has emotional stress, the sleeping suffers. Interestingly, I show a homozygous SNP for this gene- worse than Becky's but sleep like a rock and have no anxiety. My father's family's history reveals mental disorders; I am sure there is a predisposition for depression here. I think an important factor in why I do not experience these symptoms I am predisposed to is that I am consistent with proper diet, supplements, and essential oil intake!

One more example is a patient taking Vit D that is not increasing/ restoring the blood values when re-tested. Often when evaluating the VDR FOK1/TAQ1 gene, we see a mutation or SNP associated with a decrease in the body's ability to absorb Vit D, without other nutritional support. Becky is heterozygous for both of these, and I am homozygous. We both take a daily maintenance dose of Vit D nutritional support.

I must state here that a co-factor not the mutated gene itself might be the source of a patient's particular problem. This requires significant dietary and lifestyle changes. Therefore, most often the individual with gene mutations must address other issues such as inflammation, poor digestion, blood sugar problems and heavy metal toxicity when addressing the SNPs. **This is the reason I recommend that ALL PATIENTS ADDRESS THESE CO-FACTORS FIRST**. REMEMBER THAT MANY OF THE GENES IN THE GENETIC REPORT ARE STILL BEING RESEARCHED SO WE HAVE LIMITED CLINICAL INSIGHT ON THEM.

This constitutes most of the lab testing I will order on patients. If I decide that any further testing needs be done, I will advise the patient. The cost of these tests is very minimal given the wealth of information they provide.

3 The American Diet: Poor Nutrition/Wrong Recommendations

The longer I am practicing, the more justification I find for the dietary recommendations I make on a daily basis. I have said it once, and I will say it again, your dietary habits will influence your health, for better or worse, more than anything else you will do. This influence is, of course, largely due to repetition. Most people eat three or more meals, including snacks, every day of their lives. However, another major reason nutrition is so important is that the body is designed to eat foods in their most basic and unadulterated state.

The reader is probably weary of hearing how unhealthy this county is. We are supposed to be the greatest super power in the world with a great economy. One would assume that this status would also include the greatest health and longevity; as I said in the last chapter, we really miss the mark on both, and must begin to treat foods more like drugs and not just as something eaten for enjoyment. Think about it: our body never says to itself "I need a quarter pounder from McDonalds." Engineered to accept only unprocessed, non GMO (genetically modified) foods, the body's immune system, usually protecting us very well, will be over taxed when the quarter pounder is eaten. Companies know that when they modify a food, there must be some or at least a trace of the "real food" in there so that the cells of our body will accept it. This principle also applies to nutritional supplements and even drugs - most of which started out as herbs. Initially, the body accepts the food or supplement that enters until it recognizes the synthetic or modified component. Therefore, the immune system must deal with this unwanted substance. Many times it is seen as a foreign invader that the body must tag for destruction. The immune system's response varies from a sensitivity to a full-blown antibody/allergen reaction, an autoimmune reaction in which the body attacks itself. Americans should all be concerned about the plethora of erroneous information on food released by regulatory agencies that guarantee huge profits for the food industry and subsequently for the pharmaceutical industry as well.

I do know however, that some gains have been made. For example, everything coconut, previously condemned for its saturated fat, is now lauded as healthful. Many feel that the medical community is "slowly coming around" to the "more natural way" of thinking about food. We must note however, that the medical community's strategy is that something better can be synthesized or invented. I remember my mother's friend's remark talking to her about additives in food. She said "better living through chemistry." I think that sums up the conventional mindset.

In this chapter I must continue to explain the problems with the American diet, the current nutritional recommendation and why certain foods should not be a diet staple. I must also point out that the soil growing our foods has only 14% of the good minerals it had in 1934. Makes one wonder when their family doctor tells a person he gets everything he needs from his diet. Actually the rest of his advice, "don't take all of those vitamin pills as they just end up in the toilet" is in fact, correct. In truth, most of the supplements on the market are garbage due to their cheap filler content.

Most food in the SAD is processed, not slightly but highly processed. Looking at the ingredient list on a food packaging label, many people wrongly assume that they must be healthful since they are allowed on the label which usually has a very long list of dangerous substances; foods usually reveals a long list of chemical additives.

First let's briefly look at the history of the diet. Our Paleolithic ancestors relied on their hunter/gatherer skills to eat wild game and plant foods requiring little or no preparation including vegetables, fruits, berries and nuts. This continued for as long as humans have been in existence or about two and a half million years. About 10,000 years ago an agricultural revolution occurred. No one is sure why this happened but many have speculated that the expanding population and the declining wild game were the main reasons. Thus the diet which was meat and vegetable based that human's evolved on was now replaced with a cereal grain based diet which was foreign to the human digestive tract. **(15)**

The Industrial revolution arrived about 185 years ago. More technology emerged to refine sugar, flours and vegetable fats. Along with this new technology came a decline of human health which would later develop into a downward spiral - pretty much what we have today in America. At present, when food is refined or processed, vitamins are stripped away and trans fats are added to ensure a longer shelf life; this has been the case for at least the past fifty years. Americans continue buying color packaged "convenience" foods that are all over the grocery store isles in warehouse - like grocery stores. To complicate matters, high fat foods such as eggs and meats were under ridiculous scrutiny with the birth of the "Cholesterol Revolution." These foods were vilified worse than today's political candidates and, as result, these non-nutritive, low-fat, non-fat, sugar free, low cholesterol, non-cholesterol foods underwent exponential growth.

When looking at the breakdown of where the calories are coming from with the SAD of today's society, a quote from Dr. Colpo says it so succinctly. "OVER THREE QUARTERS OF THE CALORIES COME FROM STAPLES THAT WERE NON-EXISTENT DURING THE PALEOLITHIC PERIOD." We have 22% from cereal grains, 3% from potatoes, 18% from sugar and other sweeteners, 17% from junk oils, 11% from dairy products, and 5% from alcohol. This leaves a mere 20% of daily caloric intake left for all of nutrient rich foods such as eggs, meat, nuts, seafood, vegetables and fruits that used to provide all our daily energy. **(16)**

Patients always ask me why grains are not as nutritional as other foods.
First of all, lacking many necessary vitamins such as ACD and B12, cereal grains are nutritionally weak and importantly, they have no essential fatty acids. In fact they have no exclusive list of nutrients- minerals or trace elements, which cannot be found in animal products or non-cereal plant foods such as vegetables, fruits or nuts. Cereal grains also contain a substance called *phylates*, known as ant-nutrients because they block the absorption of calcium, zinc, iron and magnesium by binding to them in the gastrointestinal tract. With today's SAD, this is the last thing that should happen! There is also another substance called *pyridoxine glucoside* which decreases the availability of B6. Research has shown that B6 from cereal grains products is absorbed with far less efficiency than with animal products; B6 is essential for the breakdown of homocysteine, an amino acid that I already mentioned that can lead to heart problems if it accumulates.

If the long standing hypothesis that cereal grains can lead to a lowering in coronary heart disease were true then why is it that only one major randomized clinical study has been performed? The results actually showed a small increase in coronary and overall mortality when subjects consumed a high wheat fiber diet versus the low wheat fiber diet?

Contrasting the nutrient void grains with the nutrient rich meats, vegetables, fruits and nuts, meat has both significantly more and a higher quality of protein. You would have to consume seven to eight slices of wholegrain bread or four to five cups of brown rice to get the same amount of protein from a three ounce porterhouse steak. Furthermore, grains are deficient in the essential amino acid *lysine*. Vegetarians think that they can just eat a combination of beans and rice to get "complete protein." Like grains, legumes have a low protein content. Four ounces of lentils, for example, has 7.75 grams of protein while a steak the same size has 21 grams. Beans and cereals are also known to be extreme gas producing foods; unfortunately one has to eat large quantities to get an adequate amount of protein.

This is a good time to discuss a protein from wheat, rye and barely known as GLUTEN. Almost everyone has heard of this protein but remain unaware of its serious risks. Many quip that it is only a passing fad or followed by the "crunchy health nut" crowd and is total unnecessary. Well, I am here to be a spoiler and tell those people that it is a serious major health threat. Dr. Tom O'Bryan, chiropractor, specializes in the problems of gluten and explains in a series of DVDs its adverse effects on our bodies. For example, the molecular structure of gluten is almost identical to that of the human thyroid gland. Thus, in patients with autoimmune thyroid, in which the thyroid gland attacks itself (Hashimotos Syndrome) gluten will cause the body to inadvertently attack the thyroid gland. Gluten is a serious no - no for anyone with thyroid problems. Research has shown that 90% of all thyroid conditions are auto-immune. The problem with the gluten in this country is that it is hybridized or GMO (genetically modified) making it unrecognizable to the body and therefore seen as an unwelcomed invader in need of a hasty assault. Lately there has been some speculation that all of the gluten sensitivity we hear about today is caused by the weed killer toxin roundup (glyphosate) sprayed on all wheat fields. Yes it is a toxin and a contributing factor but we also cannot deny that today's GMO hybridized wheat shows little resemblance to that of yesteryear and consequently is not recognized by our bodies. Dr. Williams, a cardiologist and author of the bestselling book *Wheat Belly*, stated that today's wheat is the "perfect poison." He explains that wheat is an 18 inch plant born of genetic research from the 60' s and 70's with a new protein known as gliadin. He said, "**Everybody, not just those suffering from wheat sensitivity,** is susceptible to the gliadin protein because it is an opiate." Thus the wheat will bind to the brain's opiate receptors and can stimulate appetite in some. His research showed that this can lead one to eat an extra 440 calories per day. Let me give you a visual on what happens when someone eats gluten. First, it is broken down by an enzyme called tissue transglutaminase into the tiny proteins gliadin and glutenin so that it becomes small enough to be absorbed by the small intestine. Meanwhile, the GALT also known as gut associated lymphoid tissue (the immune system in the gut) will screen these proteins for potential dangers. When a person has no sensitivity to gluten, the food gets absorbed. Again keep in mind, however, that wheat today is hybridized in order to be drought and pesticide resistant. Thus, its proteins are unrecognizable by the body so they are attacked; systemic inflammation is the result.

Let me digress for a minute. There are different classifications of ways in which gluten can affect someone. A person can have a food reaction to gluten signifying a mild to moderate aversion resulting in a stomach ache or headache that is not severe or immediate. Symptoms could occur anywhere from two hours three days and seem unrelated. Good luck trying to tie these two occurrences together. For those suffering from an all - out gluten allergy, in which the throat could close and the person could die, there is automatic IGE mediated response. This is an anaphylactic reaction. Next we have food sensitivities in which the immune system is not involved and again the symptom seems totally unrelated such a headache. There is also the big daddy of all or Celiac's disease, an autoimmune disease in which the body attacks the small intestine when wheat is eaten. The problem with Celiac's is that it is EXTREMELY UNDERDIAGNOSED TODAY!!!!!!!! There is the genetic predisposition when the HLA-DQ8 and DQ2 genes are present. Currently it is thought that 35-50% of the population have these genes yet the medical establishment estimates that only 2-4% of the population have Celiac's. The problem with gluten, not generally discussed by the media is a condition known as enteropathy which literally means diseased intestines. These become inflamed and the hair-like particles or villi on the borders of the intestines cannot perform their important job absorbing nutrients from food eaten. Traditionally, Celiac's is diagnosed with a biopsy of the small intestine. However, new research discovered positive diseased intestines in patients without the HLA-DQ2 or DQ8 genes present and that 1/3rd of those with gluten sensitivity had intestinal disease. Here is a very scary statement: The British Medical Journal stated in 1999 that 87.5% of those with both a genotype (had the genes) and a positive biopsy for enteropathy had no symptoms. With symptoms, a mere 12.5% of those were diagnosed Celiac's. **The journal of Gastroenterology stated in 2001 that there are eight unconfirmed cases of Celiac's without any gastrointestinal symptoms for every one**

case of diagnosed Celiac's with intestinal symptoms. A major problem with this " silent" Celiac's disease is that those people will eat wheat without caution and really do damage to their bodies. In fact the greatest mortality with Celiac's disease has been shown to be from malignancies developed by silent Celiac patients.

After eating todays mutated wheat, the body reacts with inflammation because 5% of this wheat is unrecognizable. The inflammatory response includes antibodies made by the body to fight the invader. A problem arises, however, because along with attacking the wheat protein, the immune system also attacks the tissue transglutaminase enzyme. This enzyme not only breaks gluten down to smaller proteins, but it also functions to bind together the intestinal border cells so nothing can get through, and to increase the surface area of the microvilli- the hairy finger like projections so nutrients can be absorbed. Thus, without the TTG enzyme, the microvilli will shrink, and the body cannot absorb nutrients. Without the tight junctions between the small intestine border cells, "leaky gut syndrome" occurs; proteins leak out into the bloodstream causing further autoimmune reactions resulting in more inflammation. This scenario should warn doctors with gluten intolerant patients to look for other auto-immune diseases. For example, someone with leaky gut eats wheat which leaks into the bloodstream and ends up in the joints where it may be mistaken for arthritis. Arguably, the recommendation by the USDA to "consume at least half of all grains as whole grains" and to " increase whole grain intake by replacing refined grains with whole grains, may have new meaning for the diligent reader.

While talking about grains, we need to look at B vitamins. Meat is the best source; vegetarians often have deficiencies here. And to repeat, <u>B vitamins are essential in the breakdown of homocysteine.</u> Meat is also the best source of *carnosine,* another amino acid which is a potent antioxidant and helps prevent damage from high blood sugar due to the formation of glycation end products. AGEs (advanced glycation end products) form when glucose binds with protein without the necessary enzyme. The cell becomes less pliable, stiffer and subject to premature damage. Meat is also the best source of creatine, another amino acid the body uses to form ATP or energy. Research has shown that even though creatine can be derived from supplements, consistent blood levels were higher when obtained from red meat.

Like meats, vegetables, fruits and nuts are anti-oxidants and nutrient powerhouses. Fruits and veggies provide a lot of Vit C, folate and carotenoids such as lycopene and lutein. Folate is otherwise known as B9 essential for the methylation or energy pathway in the body as well as nerve health. Lutein is another great antioxidant for normal eye function, and lycopene aids in cancer prevention and blood vessel health. Research has discovered thousands of helpful compounds collectively known as *phytonutrients*. One in particular, polyphenols, was even far more effective as a free radical scavenger than the anti-oxidant Vit C.

It makes no difference to simply agree that green leafy veggies are nutritious if you do not plan to eat them! USDA researchers found in a 2003-2004 study that on average Americans ate 1.5 cups of vegetables daily, about 50% of the recommended daily servings. Sadly, though, more than half came from potatoes and tomatoes and only 10% came from dark green and orange vegetables. **(17)** The other low antioxidant foods which are the most commonly consumed fruits and veggies in the American diet are iceberg lettuce, French fries, bananas and orange juice.

The antioxidant content of grains is low offering nothing higher than 1 mmol/100 grams. In fact, according to Dr. Colpo, "white flour from wheat and rice, the two most commonly eaten staples in the world, possess some of the poorest antioxidant values."

The USDA dietary recommendations, since 2011, are no longer on a food pyramid; now they are on a food "plate?" With sodium they recommend, " Reduce daily sodium intake to less than 2300 milligrams (mg) and further reduce intake to 1,500 mg among persons who are 51 and older and those of any age who are African Americans or have hypertension, diabetes, or chronic kidney disease. The 1,500 mg recommendation applies to about half of the U.S. population, including children and the majority of adults. **(18)**

The SAD recommendations, which constantly urged us to consume copious amounts of non-fat or low-fat milk, whole grains and low saturated fats, and the low sodium diet has been proven ineffective. The country's health statistics substantiate this statement.. The low sodium diet was seen as a cause of high blood pressure leading to a heart attack and stroke. Remember Dr. Marshall's term, "white death" —white table salt; stripped of any nutrients it once possessed in its natural state, it now has no nutritional benefits. After unrefined salt is mined as a substance called "brine," a combination of water and salt, harmful chemicals are then added to mechanically evaporate the minerals which are then sold to stores and used in industry. Thirty nine percent sodium and sixty nine percent chloride and also a small percent of chemicals such aluminum silicate, ammonium citrate, sugar dextrose, and a trace of iodide are what is left from this process. Like grains and refined white flour, salt was originally refined to ensure shelf life. With no beneficial minerals it can sit there lifeless indefinitely. Another reason for its refinement was its dull grey color; the new brilliant white color of refined salt is more appealing to the buyers therefore bleach was in order. It was also thought that if the salt was mined from an area where there were toxins, they would be removed through this evaporation process: a chemical for a chemical, if you will. Finally, they thought if iodine was added, it would help with the goiter patients by stimulating the thyroid and adrenal glands. All of these reasons are ludicrous; just consider the 80 plus minerals in naturally mined sea salt. I must also mention the nickel grates used to sift the refined salt adding to heavy metal toxicity. In evaluating the USDA recommendation of whether a low salt diet is healthy we must consider that the research does not support it. Dr. David Brownstein, an expert on salt and the author of several books including *Salt Your Way To Health* argues, "When looking at an entire population, a low salt diet is not effective at significantly lowering the blood pressure." He goes on to state that those with diagnosed high blood pressure following a low sodium diet only lowered their blood pressure 4.9 mm systolically (the upper number) and 2.6 mm diastolically (the lower number). Here is the kicker however, those who went on low sodium diets also exhibited a huge increase in heart attacks, hormonal imbalances, and increased toxicity. In another study, of 3.000 people with high blood pressure cited by Dr. Brownstein, there was an increase in heart attacks by 430% in the group with the lowest salt intake versus the highest intake. The low salt adverse cardiac event problem can be further exacerbated by an increased activity in two kidney hormones, in aldosterone and angiotensin which will try to retain or hold on to any salt they can. This will heavily stress the nervous system and then the heart. The mineral magnesium, stripped away in refined table salt, is also crucial to maintain blood pressure. We must look at Bromine, a toxic element that will accumulate in the body if iodine levels are not maintained. Refined salt, devoid of iodine, lets this toxin build up in the body.

Another major problem with refined salt and the SAD, for that matter, is maintaining the proper pH, which is in essence a determination of the body's mineral status. This should run anywhere from 6.2-7.4. The S.AD causes most people's pH to become to acidic, as well as a mineral deficient growing soil will hasten this acidic process; an acidic pH is not good and will be a perfect environment for chronic diseases like cancer to flourish. Without adequate calcium, or an alkaline pH above 6.4, the body will simply leach it from the bones also adversely affecting the red blood cells which are manufactured by the bone marrow. This leaching is called microcrystalline hydroxyappetite and usually occurs during the night when the body is trying to heal. Then between about 5-7 am the body will redeposit this calcium into areas having affinity for it such as the ears, eyes, and some joints.

The next recommendation by the USDA is to consume less than 300 mg of daily dietary cholesterol. Despite all of the studies supporting cholesterol's job as a super antioxidant, it is still the Rodney Dangerfield of the nutritional world - it gets no respect. **Let me be clear that I am not talking about those few with inherited, extremely high, cholesterol levels who may not respond to natural treatment methods.** Cholesterol is both an alcohol and a lipid or fat, 80% of which is made by the liver; and is VITAL to cell membrane permeability or what comes and goes in and out of the cells. It makes the cells pliable unlike plastic-hydrogenated fats which make the cell membranes rigid and unable to perform necessary life functions. Hormones made in the body begin with the basic ingredient CHOLESTEROL! It is also very important in the nervous system, acting as insulation allowing for nerve transmission. Trying to disprove the benefits of cholesterol, with the use of cholesterol lowering drugs, researchers actually found that those patients had depression, cognitive decline, and motor skill reduction. You could not live without cholesterol, period. In the seventies, researches used questionable and contradictory evidence to sway the American people on the evils of cholesterol. Too much money has been invested and too many profits garnered for giant pharmaceutical companies to accept any evidence contradicting their claims and to stop selling the drugs. Think about the following statement in terms of dietary cholesterol. If you have a proper functioning metabolism, eating foods containing high cholesterol will not raise your cholesterol values. **Those with high cholesterol values must address possible clogging problems in the liver and gallbladder so that the cholesterol can do its job and then be excreted with the feces.**

The USDA recommends **only 10% of calories from saturated fats**. They also recommend monsaturated and polyunsaturated fats replace any saturated fat over the 10%. Some chemistry is in order here. Saturated and unsaturated fats differ in their chemical structure. Saturated fats are solid at room temperature, whereas unsaturated fats are liquid. Also, saturated fats have no double bond between molecules meaning there are no gaps; therefore the fat is saturated with hydrogen molecules. Conversely, unsaturated fats have double bonds which break up the chain of hydrogen molecules and create gaps allowing the fat to liquefy at room temperature. Saturated fats have gotten a bad rap due to their "presumed" association with "plastic fats" which are trans fats. Because spoilage has always been a huge problem for the food industry, they needed first to add chemicals for longer shelf life and second to cook the fat for six hours at 380 degrees, artificially hydrogenating it. They changed the molecular configuration from *cis* to *trans* making this saturated fat one carbon away from being plastic! Because the human body is constantly regenerating, creating new cells, it absolutely requires nutritious and quality foods as ingredients to make new cells. If the only ingredients the body has to create new cells are junk/inadequate, what kind of cell quality is likely to result? The outer layer of every cell is composed of fat known as the lipid layer. Consider how often cells must be replaced; there is a new gastro-intestinal lining every two or three days, (That is a very fortunate considering the SAD), a new liver every 8 weeks, and a new skeleton every year or so. Because the cells must continue to perform their trillions of functions every day, if they are not adequately formed, or sub - par, their performance will suffer greatly. As I often tell patients riddled with spinal arthritis for example, that "structure dictates function." **Following USDA recommendations on dietary fat intake, one is at risk of having worn out organs and the chronic diseases that develop from them.**

When you cook with oils for example, coconut oil, is a saturated fat- very stable and does not become rancid easily; it is the best choice for cooking. On the other hand, polyunsaturated fats have three double bonds with a high amount of unsaturation, are very unstable and break down more easily. I call polyunsaturated oils "junk oils," a label coined by Dr. Marshall, because due to this instability they become rancid as soon as they hit the digestive tract. Because of this rancid state, Dr. Marshall noted, leftovers cannot remain fresh and taste stale. Examples of polyunsaturated fats, none of which are recommended for cooking, are vegetable oil, sunflower, and the worst of all, canola oil.

Shockingly, years ago, canola oil was known as rapeseed oil and used mainly for refinishing furniture. Very inexpensive, it is used almost exclusively by restaurants. There is no fruit or vegetable called a "canola"; it is genetically engineered. Believe it or not, this oil started out as an INDUSTRIAL LUBRICATING OIL NOT MEANT FOR HUMAN CONSUMPTION. Derived from the mustard family and considered a poisonous toxic weed, it is very inexpensive to grow and harvest and insects will not eat it! Canadian growers paid the FDA 50 MILLION dollars to have rapeseed registered as "SAFE." (Source: *Young Again* and others) Some studies have shown a casual involvement in lung cancer.

Considering the American public eats in restaurants extremely frequently and consume their canola oil, some scientific animal studies are relevant. One of these studies published in a Swedish medical journal, found rapeseed "has a growth retarding effect in animals." Erucic acid, a chief component of rapeseed oil, is considered the etiology; other researchers explain the culprit is the low ratio of saturated to monsaturated fatty acids. Usually only trace amounts of erucic acid is found in the body; except when ingested in the diet as rapeseed oil, however, it is found in organ fat. It has been shown to cause fatty infiltration in heart muscle, and long term fibrosis. Respiratory capacity is diminished proportionally to the amount of dietary erucic consumed. **(19)**

Here is the kicker; Rapeseed has been shown to have a cumulative effect, taking about ten years for symptoms to appear due to its interference with normal enzyme function necessary for proper metabolism. Since it is a trans-fatty acid, it's a carcinogen. I will leave this discussion on rapeseed-canola oil with this sobering thought: in his book *Young Again*, John Thomas describes that twelve years ago in Europe and England, cows, sheep and pigs fed rapeseed oil later went blind and began attacking people. After the removal of the oil from their diet the animals displayed normal behavior?

On the other hand, olive oil is a monsaturated fat that is very beneficial for everybody. Because almost saturated, and having only one double bond, it also has a high degree of stability. You can cook with olive oil safely; it's smoke point (this is the point at which it breaks down and becomes carcinogenic) is 410 degrees if extra virgin, pure and unrefined is used.

Dr. Jerry Tennent, in his book I have been referring to, offers a good analogy to demonstrate how much saturated versus unsaturated fats a person should consume each day. He compares body cell membranes to a person's house. Everyone wants his house strong and solid with firm walls and with necessary windows and doors for entrances and exits. If the house is built with concrete blocks without windows or doors it will not be livable; nobody will be able to get in or out. Conversely, if the house consists mostly of windows, a storm will knock it down. Dr. Tennent writes, "In cells, saturated fats are strong, and unsaturated fats are porous. You need saturated fat (animal fat, for example) to make strong walls, and unsaturated fats (fish oils for example) for doors and windows." I agree with the Doctor's recommendation that the diet should contain four times as many saturated as unsaturated fats. To continue the house analogy that would mean four times as many bricks as windows and doors. **(20)**

Many readers may be confused by this last statement because of the prevalent misconception that saturated fat is bad. However, remember that trans-hydrogenated fats, previously discussed, are extremely healthy. TRANS-HYDROGENATED FATS ARE NOT SATURATED FATS.

Contradictorily, the medical textbooks stress that animal and vegetable fats are needed to act as carriers for fat soluble vitamins such as A,D,E AND K, but in the same breath, they vilify saturated fats for causing an increase in heart disease caused by high CHOLESTEROL. Dr. Tennant rightly argues that "cholesterol is presented as the villain of the civilized diet." That is so true. REMEMBER, THE RAW INGREDIENT FOR HORMONE MANUFACTURE BY THE BODY IS CHOLESTEROL. Furthermore, the liver is the body's filtering system. If left alone the liver makes as much cholesterol as it needs. Why should anyone prevent the liver's ability to clean itself and to limit hormone production by giving cholesterol lowering drugs? That reminds me of an oxymoron I often see on a commercial. They tell the middle aged man to kick his sex drive in gear and boost his "male performance" in the bedroom and the gym by rubbing testosterone cream under his arm. The commercial fails to tell the viewers that most men that age are also on cholesterol lowering drugs which decrease hormone production such as testosterone. It is like like wearing rain boots with holes in them or trying to fill a bucket with holes: both exercises in futility!

Aside from the Framingham study, one study that most experts mention considering the cholesterol/saturated fat consumption leading to stroke and heart attack, is the "The Lipid Research Clinics Coronary Primary Prevention Trial." The researchers found a 19% - 25% lower incidence in coronary heart disease compared to the placebo group. It is important to note here that the subjects were already on a low cholesterol, low saturated fat and were given cholesterol lowering drugs for the trial. Now here is where the obfuscation comes in. The study fails to mention that non heart related deaths such as strokes, cancer, violence and suicide increased compared to the placebo group. The study was heralded as a huge success by the press and medical journals. They said, the study proved that animal fats are the cause of CHD (coronary heart disease). Because this is such a highly controversial topic, independent researchers were brought in and found no statistical difference in the coronary death rate between the test subjects and the placebo group. **(21)**

It is time to mention the French paradox. Many people have always wondered why the French cuisine, noted for its high fat sauces and gravies, seems to have no effect on the population's mortality rate from CHD. In fact, France has a death rate from CHD more than 50% less than that of the United States. The Gascony region in France has a death rate is 25% of that in this country! Importantly, French cooking is full of animal fats such as eggs, meat, cheese, pates and creams. Again, some chemistry is in order here. Remember, fats do not make you fat. Along with **trans-plastic-hydrogenated fats**, **excess sugar makes you fat.**

We must look at the triglyceride molecule. It has three fatty acid chains with three glycerin; this is what most fats in our bodies are comprised of as well as the fats we eat. Triglycerides in the blood have been linked to cardiovascular disease but there is an important distinction to be made here. <u>The harmful triglycerides are not formed directly from dietary fats but are made by the liver when there are excess sugars which have not been burned</u>. **This is from the SAD full of sugary refined carbohydrates.** While I previously discussed the chemistry of carbons and hydrogens in relation to saturated to unsaturated fats, I must expand upon this. A monounsaturated fat is a fatty acid containing carbons that have one double bond between them because it lacks two hydrogens. Oleic acid is the monounsaturated fatty acid found in most of our foods and the main ingredient in olive oil. We also have fatty acids with two or more pairs of double bonds known as polyunsaturated fatty acids. Here there are at least four hydrogen molecules missing. The most common in most of our foods is linoleic acid also known as omega 6 fatty acid. An example of a three carbon double bond which is missing six hydrogen molecules is linolenic acid also known as omega 3 fatty acid. **I only mention the number of bonds and hydrogens to emphasize how stable the fatty acid is.** THE MORE SATURATED THE FAT, THE MORE STABLE IT IS. Now it is important to remember that all fats, both plant and animal are a combination of oleic, linoleic and linolenic fatty acids. Animal fats are 50% saturated while coconut oil, from a tropical plant, is 92% saturated. I would like to note that beef, for example, is only 50% saturated if from a grass fed cow. **If not and the cow is fed the usual soybean and corn diet, it will be more unhealthy, unsaturated fat**-<u>VERY BAD.</u>

Let's look at the differences between fatty acids and their chains; they are classified by researchers as having short, medium, long and very long chains. Butter and coconut are classified as short and medium chains in which there are 4 to 12 carbon atoms. Beef fat is an example of a long chain fatty acid in which there are 14 to 18 carbon molecules. Then lastly, there are very long chain fatty acids containing 20- 24 carbons, an example is fish oils.

If we look at some of the properties of these fatty acids we can see some differences setting them apart. Oleic, linoleic and linolenic fatty acids all have 18 carbons making them long chain fatty acids. For example, this would include olive oil and other polyunsaturated fats and vegetable oils.
Short and medium chain fatty acids are not absorbed by the lymph system and thus do not need to be acted upon by bile during digestion as the longer chains do. According to Dr. Tennant, "these short chain fatty acids are absorbed directly through the portal vein to the liver" and thus "supply

quick energy." Coconut and butter are short-medium chain fatty acids which, do not cause weight gain due to their portal vein direct absorption as much as olive and other vegetable oils. **It is the longer chain fatty acids, mostly oleic and linoleic, which are stored in body fat.** Another important characteristic of the short and medium chain fatty acids is the anti-fungal properties they possess for the intestinal tract as well as the anti-tumor properties that strengthen the immune system. The body uses the longer chain fatty acids to build cell membranes as well as vital hormones and also uses them to create action potentials to manage electric currents. Remember, however, the longer chain fatty acids are harder to digest and require bile salts - not good for a gallbladder functionally deprived patient, or in some cases actually gallbladder deprived! And remember, along with the weight gaining affinity with the long fatty acid chain, the very long fatty acids - most notably, the polyunsaturated, will stimulate tumor growth if eaten in excess. Again this is the modus operandi of the SAD.

I know I am going to be repeating some of this information but it will help the reader remember its importance. The SAD and the USDA recommendations, as I have earlier stated, limit the **wrong** fat in the total dietary amount allowed. Today's researchers advocate about a 3:1 - 4:1 ratio of omega 6 to omega 3 essential fatty acids. Americans far exceed this, eating upwards of 20 or 30 : 1, with polyunsaturated fat consumption up to 30% of the total caloric intake. When excess omega 6 polyunsaturated fatty acids are consumed, this interferes with crucial enzyme functioning needed to produce longer chain fatty acids. These larger chains then produce hormones vital for cellular function. Far too much inflammation, a decreased immune function, gastrointestinal irritation and high blood pressure can result from eating too many omega 6 fatty acids and insufficient omega 3s. When injured, the body needs the omega 6s for their inflammatory response necessary for healing. With the current, excessive consumption of omega 6s, however, in the SAD one could easily see that too much inflammation along with the other negative health effects I just described above can also lead to future health problems like stroke and heart attacks - the very conditions this type of eating recommendations are supposed to protect us from? *Sounds like the contraindications on a drug commercial to me.*

Another problem with polyunsaturates is the inherent instability in their in processing. Because of this they are not recommended for cooking. The unsaturation exposes these oils to becoming polymerized; they will bond not only with each other but also with other molecules. Unless the carbons are saturated with hydrogens they become unstable. This a paradox; the body needs a certain amount of essential fatty acids it cannot make on its own yet these acids are unstable and could cause much harm when oxidizing or breaking down. This creates a free radical instability in which one cell robs another of an electron, causing a domino effect which jeopardizes the DNA of the cells. Free radical damage has been associated with everything from wrinkles to autoimmune diseases such as arthritis, cancers and neurodegenerative diseases like parkinson's.

With Omega 3s it is very important to consider the degree of purity, especially in the way they are processed. Molecular distillation, used by many companies, requires such high temperatures that all of the valuable triglycerides are lost. Conversely, when not using distillation, many natural fish oils contain dangerous amounts of mercury. Some other methods remove toxins using extremely high temperatures with solvents such as hexane, damaging to Vitamins A and D absorption leading to oxidation and free radical formation. (I know this is confusing, but I will make recommendations and clarify this in a later chapter).

The guidelines then tell us to "keep trans fatty acid consumption as low as possible by limiting foods that contain synthetic sources of trans fats, such as partially hydrogenated oils, and by limiting other solid fats. I previously also explained that the trans fats in question are a man - made food processing disaster; one carbon away from plastic. The food industry loves these trans fats, like margarine solid at room temperature, because they are much cheaper than butter fat or coconut oil and their use translates into much longer shelf life. Besides margarine, most baked goods like cookies and pies contain them as well as many potato chips and microwaveable popcorn - a carcinogen because of the dangerous cooking package. Interestingly, you cannot fool animals. In a recent study animals were presented with two hamburgers, one real and one GMO. None of the animals would eat the GMO McDonalds's hamburger and even after six months to one year the hamburger did not spoil! These trans fats have negative effects on the body because it can't break them down, although it keeps trying, they remain in body fat for long periods of time. The body has to also encapsulate these acids, wasting precious energy needed to keep itself running efficiently, and try to remove them with cholesterol after it has done its job. Thus research has found that these trans fats raise the LDL cholesterol levels and lower the HDL cholesterol levels leading to stroke, type 2 diabetes and heart attack for those who consume them. The FDA has mandated that all trans fats must stop being added to foods by 2018. **(21)** This is a step in the right direction but unfortunately the USDA thinks that saturated fats, which have replaced these trans fats and have become more common in some foods, also raise levels of "bad cholesterol" and are not good for us. I am afraid with that statement they are still woefully inaccurate!

Reducing the intake of calories from solid fats and added sugars is the next recommendation. I already thoroughly explained fats so let's now focus on the sugars. We should also combine the next statement with this one: **limit the consumption of foods that contain refined grains, especially refined grain foods that contain solid fats, added sugars and sodium**. Again, we will just focus on the sugars because I have not addressed that topic yet.

Sugar; it tastes so good but in excess it is so deadly! Our bodies turn everything we eat into glucose, a form of sugar, however, a delicate blood sugar balance must be maintained. On average Americans eat in excess of 150 pounds of sugar each year! The sad truth is that many people I talk to and try to council on the dangers of excess dietary sugar constantly state "I do not eat candy or sweets." I remind them of a recent study now generally accepted that proved white bread turns to sugar faster than a snickers bar. Yes, you read it right. When researchers tested the subjects' blood an hour after eating, those who ate the bread had a higher level of glucose than those who ate the candy bar. People have to stop kidding themselves. **Most, if not all processed foods are going to contain a lot of sugar.** At least with a candy bar, one treats oneself once a week or so. It is the repetition that leads to chronic diseases. When you wake up and eat that cold breakfast cereal or toast you are eating a lot of sugar. Even if you do not add teaspoons of sugar to your tea or coffee but eat mostly processed carbohydrates such as sticky buns, donuts, muffins and cereals, you are eating too much sugar. When I say chronic diseases can result from too much sugar, I am mostly referring to adult onset type 2 diabetes and neurodenerative diseases such as Alzheimer's, and Parkinson's. Sugar is a neurotoxin and together with a protein molecule forms something called AGEs (this has become the new buzz word) or advanced glycation end products. Again, we must all keep in mind that your body turns the food we eat into glucose, a form of sugar. If eaten in moderation, sugar is tolerated by the body but it is not supposed to be a staple in our diet. The problem is, however, Americans eat WAY TOO MUCH OF IT. **In excess amounts, sugar is metabolic poison!** I always hear patients say to me, "I don't eat sweets, so why am I so heavy?" I ask them what they eat in a day and here is their reply. "For breakfast I eat a muffin or donut and two cups of coffee with one teaspoon of sugar and skim milk, or some type of creamer. For lunch I eat a sandwich with some type of meat and mayonnaise. I also eat some fruit with it and a Coke or Pepsi - usually diet. Then for supper I eat a frozen dinner or a few slices of pizza. For dessert I eat a fat free fudge bar or some other type of fat free frozen dessert. I usually snack with some pretzels or chips at night and a couple beers or glasses of wine." What is wrong with that menu? First off, it is mostly starchy carbs loaded with sugar. There is sufficient fat content, but it's the hydrogenated/trans fat dangerous kind. The most important omission with this diet is NO GREEN VEGETABLES to scavenge all of the free radicals the other foods are creating, or to help naturally detox all the heavy metals and toxic chemicals we are all exposed to on a daily basis. This patient does not have to even eat candy bars because there is a huge amount of sugar in her totally processed food diet. Soda pop has 7-8 teaspoons of sugar in one 12 ounce can; frozen dinners are loaded with sugar, as are muffins, frozen desserts and breads. Don't forget about the bread turning to sugar faster than the snickers bar experiment. Last but not least, there are no organic foods suggesting that harmful pesticides and toxic chemicals are present.

Since I already talked about the other two components of white death, white salt and in my previous book white flour, let me discuss in more detail this white sugar or third component – **because I believe it is the number one cause of most chronic diseases Americans are suffering from today.**

The two most common types of sugar are sucrose (table sugar) and high fructose corn syrup. These two are very similar chemically each containing half glucose and half fructose. As I previously stated, everything we eat is converted by the body into glucose for energy. In the early 1900's by eating fruits and vegetables, a person would get about 15 grams daily. If you contrast that today with the sugary drink concoctions, sweet rolls, and never ending dessert bars consumed, you reach a staggering 75 grams per day! These grams of sugar also consist of empty calories, meaning there is no nutritional value with their ingestion like the fiber obtained from eating fruits and vegetables. Eating all of those non-fat or low fat desserts, thinking you are doing yourself a huge favor, at the same time attempting to lose weight, consider that most if not all of those fat calories are replaced by SUGAR. Over half of the sweeteners used in today's food processing are made from corn. **(22)** Like trans-hydrogenated fatty acids**,** a man - made sugar concoction came about in the 1970's known as HFCS (high fructose corn syrup). This was "invented" to lower the cost of manufacturing processed foods substantially and to prolong shelf life. Contrary to popular belief by many even in the dietary community, all sugars are not created equal or, more importantly, are not processed the same by the body. HFCS for example, has a sweetness which is **20x** sweeter than table sugar. **(23)** I must mention the glycemic index (GI) here because many people are confused by that phrase; it is a measure of how fast the food will turn to sugar in the blood after eaten. The higher the number, the faster it will turn to sugar after ingested. This GI ranges from 1 to 100. **HIGH FRUCTOSE CORN SYRUP HAS A GLYCEMIC INDEX OF 120.** This means that when you eat this your brain thinks it is eating an overload of sweetness and to process this it releases more insulin in an attempt to get the sugar out of the blood and into the cells. Obviously, your pancreas will be working harder to keep up which eventually may lead to type two adult onset sugar diabetes. High fructose corn syrup is mostly found in all processed foods. Some examples are baked goods, salad dressings and SODA. It has been a huge money maker for the corn industry since its inclusion in our diet for the past forty years. The FDA has had it listed as generally regarded as safe or GRAS. Now, however, with the plethora of data showing the adverse dietary effects, the medical community can no longer support its incredibly excessive use.

The last dietary guideline is: **"If alcohol is consumed, it should be consumed in moderation - up to one drink per day for women and two drinks per day for men - and only by adults of legal drinking age."** There have been many studies on alcohol over the years which support this. If you look at alcohol however, you must keep in mind that in excess it is a poisonous substance that the body attempts to process quickly, excreting it with minimal incidence. An example of this poisonous effect is the drunken college kid who actually reaches "black out" status to be carted off in an ambulance to the local hospital emergency room; his stomach is pumped to avoid death by alcohol poisoning. Many students become unconscious before the body can process the alcohol. Since the liver produces an ounce of alcohol as a by - product of cleansing the body on a daily basis, I agree that one to two drinks per day may not be dangerous for an otherwise unburdened body. If it lowers stress which in turn lowers your blood pressure and racing heart beat etc., then maybe it is acceptable for most people to drink in moderation. We also cannot forget, however, that alcohol turns to sugar in the blood stream very quickly and is also a dehydration inducer just like caffeine. In fact, one gets hung over from alcohol due to the meninges, coverings on the skull, which shrink because of the dehydration.

Speaking of caffeine, a drug, I must talk about detrimental effects of its excessive use, on the body; raising blood pressure, interfering with normal sleeping patterns, causes a rapid heartbeat, seizures and addiction to boot. A less severe but chronic insidious problem with excess caffeine consumption is dehydration. With every 8 ounces of caffeine consumed, a person needs to drink 32 ounces of water to make up for the water necessary to process it. (This is a very profound statement that I may have already made or may make again). If a person drinks two cups of coffee a day, they need at least 64 ounces to prevent dehydration. Another huge problem in this country with caffeine is energy drinks. They can have up to 500mg of caffeine in them. The average American consumes about 200 mg of caffeine per day. One cup of coffee has about 85 mg of caffeine in it. You can see that this country consumes too much caffeine whether it be from coffee or energy drinks.

The guidelines recommend that we "increase intake of fat-free or low-fat milk and milk products, such as milk, yogurt, cheese, or fortified soy beverages." This statement is so BLATENTLY WRONG THAT IS SICKENS ME. Fat free is NEVER good because it means altering mother nature's ingredients and normal fatty acids. I previously explained, in detail, that fat-free and lower fat means more sugar and other fillers to make up for the fat. I realize that many readers, and also some of my patients love milk, and believe me that I have my share of farmers as patients and I am not making any friends in the farming community with my next statement. A great many humans are allergic to cow's milk; in fact dairy products cause 85% of food sensitivities. Let's focus on cow's milk, however, since the guidelines endorse it. A cow's milk is meant to make a cow reach 1000-1200 pounds in one year. IMPORTATNTLY, it is for cows not humans. To accomplish this, milk contains the growth hormone IGF 1 (insulin growth factor). Unfortunately, this mimics the IGF 1 in humans; therefore, when we drink cow's milk, it causes our bodies to release sugar into the cells at a much greater rate than normal, increasing the chances of obesity and diabetes. In addition, many cows receive Bovine Growth Hormone which magnifies the IGF by 80%.

One glass of cow's milk is legally allowed to have 135 pus cells in it. Yuck. Cow's milk not only has a huge amount of active hormones and scores of allergens, but also has measurable quantities of toxic chemicals such as pesticides and herbicides, blood, feces, viruses, bacteria and up to fifty antibiotics. Furthermore, anything the cows eat will be in their milk; some cow's milk has even tested positive for radioactive fallout from nuclear missile testing. Another alarming fact brought to my attention by Dr. Lonnie Herman, is that many cows actually carry Bovine Leukemia which can be passed on to their offspring through their milk. The large milk producing states like Wisconsin statistically have much higher rates of human leukemia - makes you wonder. Another disease passed to the cow's offspring is Johnne's disease which has symptoms similar to Crohn's: gas, bloating, uncontrollable diarrhea, gut lesions, and abscesses.

It is estimated that 60% of Wisconsin's residents would test positive for Johnne's disease. You have to ask, how many people have contracted Crohn's from infected cows?

For many people the main milk protein, casein, is toxic and can cause eczema, acne, kidney problems, arthritis, tooth decay, irritable bowel or Crohn's, colitis and multiple sclerosis. The digestive complaints people usually describe from milk and dairy products are mainly from digesting the sugar lactose. Remember, kids with recurrent ear infections are twice as likely to suffer from dairy/milk allergies. WHEN TAKEN OFF DAIRY PRODUCTS MOST KIDS' SYMPTOMS WILL GREATLY IMPROVE.

Cheese and yoghurt contain milk and, therefore, the same warnings apply. However, most people do not consume as much cheese as they drink milk and the yoghurt is fermented, which is actually good for the digestive tract - if no sugar is added of course.

This brings me to the USDA recommendations on soy. First, look at how soy is processed in the United States. The soybean is separated into protein and oil, neither of which is safe or natural when eaten by humans. Ninety percent of soy is GMO, according to Dr. Mercola, because like wheat, growers want soy to be resistant to the infamous pesticide, Roundup. Therefore, GMO introduces a new bacterium into our food supply. Studies show that the gene inserted into the GMO soy can get into human cell DNA and continue to function long after it is eaten, thereby continuing to produce allergic proteins in the gut. WOW. Again, like wheat and dairy, this will cause the body to attack it and with that comes all of the annoying immune response (allergy type) symptoms. Some Russian studies have also shown potential infertility in future generations. Soy also contains "anti-nutritional factors" which interfere with enzymes needed to digest protein. Some of these factors include saponins, soyatoxin, phylates, oxalates, goitrogens and estrogens; the fact that soy is estrogenic or has estrogen like qualities adds to its pernicious effects. Young boys who consume a lot of soy could succumb to gynecomastia - an enlargement of the breasts; woman consuming a lot of soy can grow fibroids. There are cases of woman who followed the soy based Medifast diet only to later need fibroid removal surgery. A problem would not arise if only taken in small quantities however. America's consumption is huge because 80% of the world's soy supply is in animal feed. I often hear the question "why do the Japanese consume so much soy without any health consequences?" There are two reasons: First, they do not consume a lot of soy in Asia using it merely as a condiment and have on average one or two tablespoons at a sitting. Secondly, they use **organic fermented** soy which is very nutritious; Americans on the other hand, consume non fermented, contaminated soy. Remember tofu is non-fermented soy and should be avoided.

The last USDA guideline I will discuss is, "**to increase the amount and variety of seafood in the diet by choosing seafood in place of meat and poultry.**" Since I mentioned GMO several times in this chapter, You can then guess my surprise when I read about a GMO fish coined "Frankenfish;" it has three chromosomes and all are female. They grow 50% larger and twice as fast as the salmon Mother Nature produces because they are given a growth hormone from the Pacific Chinook Salmon, combined with a gene from an eel - like fish called the Ocean Pout. The result is year around growth rather than growth in only part of the year in the natural fish. A news reporter sat down to a meal with both the normal salmon and the GMO salmon, and found no difference in taste or texture. The producers said that the Frankenfish are sterile but admitted that some will probably escape their fish farm enclosures and breed with the wild salmon. This is both very serious and scary because most restaurants do not have to list what kind of salmon they are serving and if, Frankenfish, the body does not recognize it like many of the GMO foods. **More ALLERGIES will result**.

4. Essential Oils

Why essential oils? **The global cost of healthcare is 6.5 Trillion dollars!** American are less healthy today than in all the preceding years and this trend continues on a steady decline despite the strives in technology and scientific research. This is puzzling to say the least? According to the National Institute on Drug Abuse, **our biggest drug problem today is not the recreational drugs but the prescription drugs.** According to Pharmacoepidemiology & Drug Safety, the number of pain killer overdoses more than tripled from 1999-2006. And with vulnerable preschool aged children now the latest target by the BIG PHARMA for cholesterol and anti-depressant medications, something must be done to stop the drug abuse.

About two years ago my wife and I decided to investigate essential oils as a way to enhance the effectiveness of treatment. Instead of synthetic medications the body cannot recognize or utilize, as well as the plethora of adverse toxic side effects and the possibility of addiction, **we need natural cost-effective solutions free from side effects and addiction.**

Essential oils have gained well deserved recognition over the past few years. Many of my current patients tell me about someone, usually a relative, who uses the oils with good effects. In fact, we were introduced to the oils by a woman who gave us some samples. We thoroughly investigated the history of the oils and the model of the company that distributes them before we decided to incorporate them into our treatment therapies. Essential oils surprisingly have been around for a very long time, centuries in fact.

Derived from aromatic plants they have been known as the most effective medicine. What exactly are they? Essential oils are the natural extracts from life protecting fluids of plants. Many people are not aware that plants have incredible protection against insects and other pathogens, stored as an oil and extracted from the plant by using a process called distillation. The ancient Egyptians and Chinese are credited as the first to use essential oils. The Egyptian document "Ebers Papyrus," written between 1553 and 1555 BC, details the use of Frankincense oils and other aromatics for certain ailments. However, the oils used in ancient Egypt were not as concentrated as today's steam distilled oils. They were a combination of animal fats and plants in which the essential oils were extracted using hot oils and are considered the precursors of today's essential oils. **(24)** It is important to remember that the Egyptians did not always distinguish between perfumes and medicines; for instance, one scented oil may serve two purposes, medicinal. and aromatic. An ancient Chinese text known as "Pen Tsao," believed to have been written in 2500 BC, explains the medicinal uses of over 300 plants; many historians believe the Chinese started studying aromatics about the same time as the Egyptians. **(25)** Moreover, Babylonians actually put essential oils in the mortar when they built their temples to ensure a constant aromatic atmosphere. This method of building temples was handed down to the Arabs who then built their mosques this way.

The Greeks actually attributed the sweet smell of aromatics to divine origin and in Roman, as well as Greek bath houses, aromatic oils were extensively used. In the fourth century BC, Hippocrates, the father of modern medicine, described that burning certain aromatic substances protected people from contagious diseases. In fact, throughout Europe from the fourteenth to sixteenth centuries, many herbal writings were published which included recipes for essential oils. Those who used aromatics were thought to be the only ones who survived the plagues that ravaged that period.
In the 1920's, however, a French cosmetic chemist named Rene Maurice Gatttefosse began the scientific study of therapeutic properties of essential oils. One day, while making perfume, he burned his arm badly. Desperately looking for some cold liquid to soak his arm in, he found a tub full of Lavender oil and immediately felt better when his arm touched the oil. More importantly, however, instead of developing into a blistering inflammatory problem, his arm healed very quickly and without any scar. Thus, the healing properties of essential oils were reclaimed. It was Gatttefosse who then coined the term "aromatherapy." **(26)** Jean Valnet MD, an army surgeon investigated natural ways for total health, wrote his first book at 44 on aromatherapy and several others on herbal medicine.

Another pioneer, Robert Tisserand, is known as the "father of modern aromatherapy." His book, *The Art of Aromatherapy* was instrumental in bringing both professional and public widespread recognition to aromatherapy. These three men paved the way for modern day usage of essential oils, however, considering the advances in modern technology and scientific breakthroughs, they may have only scratched the surface of their broader use.

There are many essential oils on the market, and unfortunately, many of the companies selling them are unscrupulous. Like with nutritional supplements, it is of the utmost importance that pure, high quality essential oils are used. **They MUST be harvested from the plant not made in a laboratory.** While still in the plant, these substances are known as essences; when liberated from the plant, they are known as essential oils. "In the true sense, essential oils are either distilled or expressed," (Arctander 1960) and there are many methods of accomplishing this. First there is water distillation in which the plant material in water is slowly brought to a boil; there is also water-steam distillation in which plant material is mixed with water and then subject to steam. In steam distillation, pressurized steam is blown through the plant material. A process known as cohobation occurs when the original mother liquid is re - introduced and re-distilled in order to recover water soluble components lost in the first run. In fractional distillation, various stages of distillation are interrupted. Dry distillation is used without any liquid or steam in a vacuum. In a process called expression, after citrus peels are scraped, the essence is collected by centrifuge. Other methods of extraction, involving dangerous chemical solvents, are too harsh for the result to be "pure essential oils."

To repeat, in order for safe effective therapeutic use of essential oils, it is imperative that they are pure. A difficulty in achieving this lies the fact that many of the so called essential oil products are listed under the general heading "essential oils" and therefore are very confusing to the average buyer with such labels as "nature identicals," "isolates," "perfume compounds" and "aromas" all reconstitutions, none of which are good, and, many of which are toxic. These synthetic compounds are resorted to in order to meet the demands of an increased market and give the synthetic uniformity that nature cannot and should not provide. The perfume industry is the largest consumer of essential oils, and depending on costs, uses mixtures containing synthetic substances to develop fragrances. **(27)** From the research my wife Becky and I have done over the past few years, the essential oil company which impressed us the most in all aspects from their sourcing method to their extraction process, to their quality testing methods, is **dōTERRA** by far. The name is a Latin derivative and means "gift of the earth." This company was started in 2008 by a group of healthcare and business professionals who shared profound, life changing experiences using essential oils and they wanted to bring a new standard of therapeutic grade essential oils to everybody that would appeal to both novices and experts in the field. They also wanted to create a new paradigm for essential oils. At first offering, dōTERRA introduced 25 single oils and 10 oil blends which were received with great accolades by experts in the field for both purity and therapeutic grade quality. Since that time there are over twice that amount. In addition to their commitment to continuous research and development of new oils and proprietary essential oil blends, dōTERRA also offers nutritional and healthy living products based on essential oil technologies.

Keeping up with the Japanese "KAIZAN" principle of constant improvement, dōTERRA recently employed a new scientific advisor, a PhD in Pharmacognosy who pioneered a new technology called "ARC PLOT," "a new and more complete testing protocol ensuring pureness of the essential oil." Up until recently, the oils had always gone through a process of initial testing, then secondary validation, then final validation. This consisted of such procedures as gas chromatography and mass spectroscopy. However, because dōTERRA strives to have the best quality and research, product innovation and sourcing, while adhering to their original mission statement, another step using the arc plot has been added. The arc plot uses one visual graph detecting any adulteration, as well as inspecting the ratios of components, and the composition of the essential oil. The graph consists of a 12 spoke spider web - like drawing in which each spoke represents a biochemically linked pair and has a different scale. If one of the above criteria for essential oil purity is not met, it will be obvious using the arc plot.

One of the most attractive parts of this company is the sourcing methods used to gather the raw plant materials needed to make the essential oils. They refer to it as co-impact sourcing; they use a global network of artisans to provide their raw materials sourcing because the company feels that where these plants are grown has a major impact on their constitution and thus its potency. By using local artisans who have grown these plants and flowers for generations, they know the growing environment maximizes the essential oil's potential. DōTERRA also realizes that by using these experienced indigenous growers, who have learned harvesting secrets over generations, that certain parts of the plant will be harvested only at specific times ensuring the highest quality of the essential oils. Moreover, and what Becky and I feel separates this company from the rest, is that they create industry for the local growers where there has been no viable industry. In other words, does not allow dubious farming and harvesting practices that rape the land by destroying future farming of the product. DōTERRA does other incredible charitable work through their nonprofit dōTERRA Healing Hands Foundation. Some of the foundation's accomplishments to date are: Nepal earthquake relief in 2015, a Guatemalan trip in 2015, trips to Bolivia and Ghana in 2014, and the Haiti water project, to name a few. They built a school on one of these trips, a medical center on another. They taught teenage girls the proper hygiene so that they could attend school with boys. Importantly, on one trip they devised a method to get fresh water daily to a village people who used to walk miles every time they needed it. We feel that it says a lot about a company's integrity to help their fellow man; **more of that selflessness is needed in today's medical community!**

The very strictly regulated process of extraction dōTERRA uses is known as low-heat steam distillation. Steam under pressure is circulated through the raw plant materials and the essential oils are liberated and taken away with the steam. The steam then cools and the oils are collected when they separate from the water. In order to maintain the proper chemical composition of the oil extract, the temperature and pressure is closely monitored and regulated.

To ensure the highest quality of the oil, dōTERRA created a third party testing company, the CPTG (certified pure therapeutic grade), for the most stringent testing protocols enforcing consistency, purity, and quality batch to batch. After distillation, the oils are immediately CPTG tested for chemical composition. Then a second round of testing is done, at their production facility, making sure what was distilled and tested is the same essential oil that was received. Next, a third review is done on the chemistry of the oil in a three phase procedure as the oils are packaged into bottles for consumption. This last check confirms the essential oil is free from contaminants and any unexpected changes during its production. The CPTG includes the following tests: Organoleptic testing, Microbial testing, Gas chromatography, Mass spectrometry, (FTIR) Fourier Transform Infrared Analysis, Chirality testing, Isotopic analysis, and Heavy metal analysis.

I want to explain the methods of using essential oils which can be divided into three categories: inhalation, topical and internal. With inhalation or aromatic use, a person inhales the oil or a vapor of volatile aromatic components that have evaporated from the oil. One could also use a nebulizing diffuser which uses room temperature air to break the oils into a micro-fine mist that is diffused into the air. There is also a ultrasonic nebulizer in which vibrations mix the water and oil into a fine vapor. This will be suspended in the air for hours improving the air quality due to the oil's antiseptic, antibacterial properties, and will remove a variety of unwanted airborne chemicals resulting in the users improved mental and physical well-being. To be the most effective, a timer can be placed on the diffuser so that the olfactory system (smell) gets a break before the next diffusing session. Research has found that the most therapeutic benefit occurs when the time interval of diffusion is every 15 minutes in a 24 hour period. The essential oils can be directly inhaled by holding the bottle up to the nose and inhaling; this is found to be the simplest way to affect moods and emotions. One could also put a few drops of oil on their hands and then inhale into the cupped hands. Moreover, one could inhale a couple of drops placed on a towel or tissue. You can also put a few drops in hot water and inhale the vapor but remember that heating the oils will take away some of the benefits. In a small area such as a vehicle, a cotton ball with drops of essential oils can be attached to an air vent or in a house on a ceiling fan. Essential oils can also be worn as perfume or cologne; one to two drops are placed on the neck, wrist or anywhere on the body. You can also mix your own simple cologne or perfume by combining 10-15 drops of essential oil with about 20 drops of alcohol and a teaspoon of spring water. **(28)**

The mechanism by which the olfactory system processes the inhaled oil is enhanced by the fact that it is anatomically closely connected to the brain's limbic system which includes structures such as the hippocampus controlling for long term memory, the amygdala for emotions, the hypothalamus regulating the autonomic nervous system and hormones and the cingulate gyrus which regulates blood pressure, heart rate and attention. Each inhalation of essential oil also creates an electro-chemical response. This impacts both the brain as well as other portions of the nervous system while simultaneously small amounts of essential oil enter your lungs to be delivered throughout the body via the bloodstream.

Essential oils can also be applied topically. They can be applied to the body's skin, hair, teeth, nails, or mouth. When applying internally to the mouth or gums please consult a professional due to the possibility of irritation. If no carrier oil, such as fractionated coconut oil, olive oil or almond oil is used with the essential oil, it is referred to as a "neat" application of the oil. One must exercise caution in topical use since some of the oils are very potent and can irritate the skin. These are often referred to as "hot" oils. With all oils, however, no matter how potent, only 1-3 drops are necessary to be effective. **More is not better when it comes to essential oil dosage**. Although less sensitive skin, the bottoms of the feet are packed with nerve endings and pores that greatly enhance their oil absorption time second only to the area behind the ears and the wrists. To feel noticeably energized, relaxed or peaceful, one can rub 3-6 drops into the bottom of each foot. To prevent excess oil from being absorbed by the body, always dilute the oil by 15-30% when massaging a large area. With infants dilute the oils with fractionated coconut oil at a 1-3 drop to 1 tablespoon ratio and for children aged 2-5, a 1-3 drop per one teaspoon ratio. Some people prefer to blend oils or make their own mixtures; remember, however, it can be dangerous depending on how the oils are made and how their chemical composition changes if improperly mixed. **Thus, it is better to layer the oils when applying them for topical use.** This consists of just applying one oil by rubbing it in and then applying another oil etc. There is no need to wait at all between each oil as they are absorbed very quickly. Bathwater is another way to topically get the benefit of essential oils. Research has shown that penetrating the skin is increased 100 fold if essential oils are added to a bath; the oil separates from the water and the skin draws it from the top of the water. Add 3-6 drop of water and then soak for about 15 minutes. The oils can also be added to a shower gel base in a ratio of 3-6 drops per ½ ounce; keep in mind, however, the oils will be more evenly dispersed and do not have a chance to separate. In another method, reflexology, oils are applied to certain points on the hands and feet. A vibrational healing energy along meridians and neurological pathways to end organs is created. The last topical method is massage. Interestingly, there are several different massage techniques that can elicit many different responses. Some elicit healing and relaxation while others are invigorating and energize the system. Furthermore, no matter what type of effect is desired, essential oils can greatly enhance the massage experience by simply combining 3-10 drops of oil with 1 tablespoon of fractionated coconut or some other carrier oil.

Internal application (ingesting) of essential oils importantly demands that only pure, therapeutic, unprocessed grade oils are used. This means those diluted or heavily processed with chemicals must be avoided. GRAS (generally regarded as safe for human consumption) is the acronym given by the U.S. FDA to some essential oils for internal use. The FDA also gives some essential oils a FL (flavoring agent) or FA (food additive) status. FL status is for essential oils added to foods to improve the aroma or quality of taste. The FA designation is for oils that are added to food used to maintain food safety, freshness and nutritional value. Some examples of essential oils designated as GRAS are cassia, ginger, helichrysum, marjoram, oregano, vanilla and ylang - ylang. Some examples of those given the FA and FL designation are dill, melaleuca, vetiver and frankincense. **Remember, not all essential oils are given the GRAS designation and are not for**

internal use. An example would be cedarwood.

There are several ways to take the oils internally. We can simply place a drop or two of the essential oil under the tongue. The absorption is almost immediate due to the shallow blood vessel supply below the tongue's surface. This method is faster and much more efficient than when swallowed since it bypasses the liver metabolism and is readily available for distribution throughout the body where needed. **(28)**

Another very common way to take oils internally is to encapsulate them in a plant based capsule. Dosage would be anywhere from 1-14 drops of one to several different oils. This capsule could also be diluted with olive oil if needed and gives the user the advantage of being "tasteless."

Drinking the oils is another way to take essential oils internally, but remember their potency will be diminished because they must go through the gastrointestinal tract and are broken down before going into the bloodstream directly. Dosage is about a drop or two of essential oils to one or more cups of water, coconut milk, rice milk or almond milk.

The last method I will discuss is cooking with the essential oils. You must keep in mind that since the oils are very concentrated, it only takes **one drop or less. In fact sometimes it is only the amount on the end of a toothpick that will be sufficient in cooking.** Recently, Becky and my daughter made guacamole and had forgotten to buy cilantro; they used a tooth pick dab of cilantro essential oil and it did the trick! Keep in mind anytime the oils are heated, their potency will definitely be adversely affected.

I must also mention safety guidelines or considerations while using essential oils. Each individual body chemistry is unique and therefore somewhat unpredictable in its response to the essential oils. Unwanted or "negative" effects are unusual with essential oils; however, it is important to understand their characteristics so that proper steps can be taken if they occur. Probably the most common unwanted effect is skin irritation or rash. The most basic test to assess body tolerance for any oil is the skin test. A drop of oil is rubbed on the surface of the skin, usually on the underside of the wrist or forearm, to determine if any redness or itchiness results after an hour. If an irritation occurs you can simply use a carrier oil such as fractionated coconut or olive oil to dilute it and usually render it useable. It is important to note however, that if an undiluted oil irritates the skin on the forearm or wrist, it is worth trying on the soles of the feet where the skin is very tough, yet the absorption rate is fast.

Another important cautionary reminder is to keep oils out of the reach of children. These oils can be considered a form of natural medicine and can be harmful if large quantities of the wrong oil are ingested. **Do not apply the essential oils directly to the eyes or the ear canals**; this includes the eyelids and rubbing around the eyes, handling contact lenses or touching the interior of the nose. Any skin around mucous membranes and the genitals will be very sensitive and prone to irritation. **Again, more is definitely not better with essential oils**. A little goes a long way. With the dōTERRA brand - I am not familiar with many of the other brands, there is a reducer in the bottles so only one drop at time comes out. High quality oils are purposefully very concentrated thus requiring very small amounts due to potency. **Wintergreen, for example, is alright in moderation but can be toxic to the liver in high doses.** Although there is a consensus among aromatherapists that topically or externally applied essential oils in normal amounts are not harmful to a developing fetus, it is recommended that pregnant woman consult with their physician prior to using any essential oils. Some breast feeding woman report that using peppermint essential oil resulted in a decrease in milk production so to err on the side of caution so to speak, **it is recommended that breast feeding woman avoid not only peppermint oil** but any blends containing peppermint oil such as Digestive Blend, Metabolic Blend and Soothing Blend. There are also the "hot" oils I talked about previously, which can be passed on through the mother's milk and can irritate the infant both with their taste and detoxification of toxins effect. **When it comes to applying essential oils to infants and children directly, care must be taken to avoid transfer of oils or cross contamination to such areas as the eyes**. To remedy this it is recommended after the oil is applied to have that area covered, until sufficiently absorbed. **Also remember that applying the essential oils to babies, young children and the elderly require more diligence than with others as their skin is more sensitive and susceptible to irritation.** There are those essential oils that **heighten or increase a person's photosensitivity to the sun increasing the chances of skin staining.** These are most notably the citrus oils such as Angelica, Grapefruit, Lemon, Lime, Orange, Tangerine, Wild Orange and Bergamot - which contains bergaptene, a dominant photosensitizer and can cause severe reactions such as rashes and even sometimes dark pigmentations. **This increased photosensitivity not only includes exposure to natural sunlight but sunlamps or any other exposure to UV rays. Thus, when using photosensitizing oils, wait at least 6 -12 hours before exposing skin to UV rays. Use extra caution with Bergamot. (29) Some serious or critical health conditions have contraindications to certain oils.** Although these condition may benefit greatly from the use of essential oils, it is recommended that a healthcare professional or aromatherapist is consulted prior to their use.

The essential oil containers are deliberately made of dark, high quality glass. Many of the oils will dissolve the plastic and it will leach into the oil. Thus when making a capsule to take internally, it is important to take the capsule immediately because the potent oils will dissolve the capsule. If you want to add a few drops of lemon oil to your drinking water, it is not recommended to use a low quality plastic bottle because of leaching; a glass or stainless steel container should be used. **Lastly, many oils are flammable so keep them away from an open flame.**

When properly used, essential oils (I am referring to dōTERRA brand that we use in my office) are safe and effective for all ages. They are 100% pure plant extracts **50-70 times more powerful than herbs with zero fillers, pesticides, chemicals or artificial ingredients**. They have no side effects and are non - habit forming. <u>**That is very hard claim to make today; try to get that from a drug company**</u>. The effectiveness of the essential oils lies in their ability to penetrate the cell's exterior, thus helping to police it. Moreover, these oils are also very economical, costing only cents per serving. One oil used to aid in digestion, Digestive Blend, for example, can aid an upset stomach only requiring three drops rubbed on the abdomen for 12 cents per drop, or a whopping 36 cents. How is that for cost effective?

Let me now discuss some of the most popular dōTERRA oils and their use. <u>Keep in mind some are single oils and some are blends named for their function</u>. **Oregano oil**: Oregano is nature's most potent anti-biotic, supports the immune and GI systems, and acts as a cleansing and purifying agent. **Digestive Blend** can sooth and ease occasional stomach discomfort and ease feelings of queasiness, when a food eaten disagrees with you. **Lavender** is widely known for its calming and relaxing qualities by helping to ease feelings of tension and can also soothe skin irritations and can even reduce the appearance of some skin imperfections.
Melaleuca is renowned for its skin cleansing and rejuvenating properties.
Respiratory Blend helps to minimize the effects of seasonal threats by maintaining the feelings of a clear airway and easy breathing. **Peppermint** relieves feelings of tension and fatigue and is an energy boost when applied to the temples. It promotes digestive health by helping to reduce gas, bloating and occasional indigestion. A natural bug repellent, it also promotes healthy respiratory function and clear breathing. **Lemon** naturally cleanses the body and is a digestive aid. It supports healthy respiratory

function and promotes a positive mood. Lemon oil is a very diverse cleaner and can be used on countertops, as a furniture polish, to clean tarnished metals and as a degreaser in hand washing. **Frankincense, the granddaddy of all oils,** promotes balanced mood, focus and relaxation.
Calming Blend promotes relaxation and restful sleep, calms emotion and lessens tension. **Joyful Blend** lessens feelings of stress and elevates mood promoting feelings of confidences, self-worth and vitality. **Protective Blend** offers a natural alternative to immune support, supports healthy respiratory function, protects against environmental threats and is an all-purpose cleaner.
Grounding Blend evokes a feeling of tranquility and balance and helps ease anxious feelings. **Metabolic Blend** is a mood enhancer promoting healthy metabolism which helps manage hunger cravings. **Tension Blend** eases stressful feelings and calms emotions. **Cellular Complex** supports healthy cell repair and regeneration, and anti-oxidant protection against the inevitable free radical attacks our bodies undergo due to oxidative stress as we age.

You should have noticed, many of the indications for use of these different oils are the same. In other words, you can take several different oils for the same benefit. This is a very beneficial since everybody's body chemistry is unique; each person may react differently to each oil. This gives you several choices among the oils for various health conditions.

Let me offer some examples of how you can boost the body's support to restore balance when it is suffering from certain health challenges. Gastrointestinal complications are very common for those over age 65 taking NSAIDS (non-steroidal anti-inflammatories). In fact 1 in 4000 die from GI complications from these over the counter drugs. Many people are looking for an alternative source for pain reduction. Some oils that support the body in its effort to fight pain are: Soothing Blend, Lavender, Oregano, Lemon, and Peppermint. For those suffering from a lot of difficult, unrelenting, pain, Marjoram or Oregano mixed with Frankincense has been highly effective and referred to as the "morphine shot." There is also a mixture of oils known as "the bomb" which aids the body in combating environmental invaders (infections). The oils are Protective Blend, Lemon, Oregano, Frankincense, and Peppermint.

There are many instances where oil blends can be used. Here, the sum is greater than its parts in terms of benefit. When someone is very anxious and needs help to calm down, Calming Blend and Grounding Blend can be a great help. As I am writing this book, dōTERRA just released its emotional aromatherapy group of oils. Modern scientific research is confirming what we have known for centuries: Emotions, the culmination of many complex psychological and sensory stimuli including olfaction, (smell) can be positively influenced by delicate complex aromatic compounds.

The Emotional Aromatherapy System " is a revolutionary organization of aromatic plant families around a continuum, of emotions for a simple, profound approach to using fragrant essential oils in emotional aromatherapy applications." This is a very easy, accessible system to help better deal with any negative emotions. There is a line of proprietary oil blends representing six categories of emotional well-being. A person simply identifies the category of negative emotions they are feeling on the emotional aromatherapy wheel diagram then selects the corresponding essential oil blend that is right for them. This may consist of more than one oil since sometimes there is more than one emotion at any given time. We have the Encouraging Blend, Uplifting Blend, Inspiring Blend, Renewing Blend, Comforting Blend, and the Reassuring Blend.

Many people are probably wondering if there is a more objective method of finding out which oil is indicated for them even though they have no symptoms. My wife and I also pondered this and began researching the "Zyto" machine. The Zyto compass is classified as a biofeedback device and works by measuring galvanic skin response in which the device detects subtle energy changes in the skin's electrical properties. A zyto scan only takes a few minutes to perform and is painless. We find this machine to be very accurate; it generates a report based on these readings telling the user how many biomarkers are out of balance. This is followed by a list of essential oils and/or supplements for that particular imbalance. The highest out of range biomarker is usually where a person should start with essential oils. Thus, the Zyto is another important tool to prioritize which oils a person needs. The list of suggested oils is advised for three months use after which another scan is recommended to assess the balance of the biomarkers.

Although, the next chapter will deal with dōTERRA's cleanse which entails the use of supplements, *Detoxification Blend* is an oil blend which naturally supports the detoxification of unwanted substances in the body by offering liver support.

From the first chapter, I am sure most readers would agree that we live in a very toxic world. I would also be willing to bet that most would opt for less toxic ways to live if they were not too intrusive. One startling fact that you probably did not know might nudge you in the right direction: **Over 100,000 kids, under the age of 6, are sickened by household cleaners each year**. Let's look at cleaning and laundry products and how easy it would be to change them. Essential oils can be mixed with other ingredients to make safe, non-toxic, effective household cleaners.

1). All-purpose cleaner: 1.5 cups of white vinegar, 2 cups of hydrogen peroxide, 10 drops of melaleuca, and 10 drops of your choice of oil depending on the effect you are after. *DōTERRA has a chart on which oils can be chosen based on the effect you want. In other words if you are looking for an antibacterial one, your choices of oils are: Thyme, Melaleuca, Geranium, Oregano, Cinnamon, Lemon, Peppermint, Rosemary, Lime, and Lemongrass. The chart also has oil choices for the following effects as well: viral and bacterial decreasing, freshening, insect preventing, and mold.* Add the selected ingredients to a 24-32 ounce spray bottle and fill with water. Shake it up and it is ready to spray.

2). Toilet bowl cleaner: ½ cup of baking soda, ¼ cup of white vinegar, and 5 drops of your choice of oils depending on what effect you are after.
Pour water into the toilet bowl until it drains. Sprinkle baking soda into the toilet bowl. Add essential oils. Scrub with a toilet brush. Pour vinegar in and scrub as needed. Let mixture sit in toilet. Close the lid to flush.

3). Furniture polish: Combine ½ cup of olive oil and 10 drops of lemon oil. Polish leather or wood with a soft cloth.

4). Carpet and upholstery freshener: Combine 20 drops of essential oil, again your choice, with 3 cups of baking soda. Cover and let mixture rest overnight. Sprinkle on carpets or upholstery to freshen and deodorize. Wait several hours or overnight. Vacuum.

5). Floor wash: Mix 1 gallon of water, ¼ cup of white vinegar, 5 drops of lemon or melaleuca and 2 drops of liquid soap in a bucket.

6). Basic laundry powder: ½ cup soap flakes or 1 bar of soap grated finely, 1 cup borax, 1 cup washing soda (not baking soda), 5-10 drops of an essential oil depending on desired effect. Combine ingredients well and store in an airtight container. Use about 2 tablespoons per load.

7). Stain remover: 2 parts hot water, 1 part baking soda, 1 part hydrogen peroxide, 1-3 drops of lemon oil. Mix the amount for one use. You can spot treat stains and allow to sit overnight; then launder as usual.

8). Fabric softener: 1 gallon white vinegar, 15-30 drops of desired essential oil. Pour essential oil into bottle of vinegar. Add this to your washer's rinse cycle.

Tips: Add 5 drops of essential oil to the detergent in your wash cycle to boost cleaning or disinfecting. Use 20 drops of Eucalyptus for dust mites.

For those of you less adventurous, who would rather not make your own cleaner or detergent, dōTERRA has you covered. They have a clear concentrate containing the Protective Blend essential oil that can be used as an all-purpose cleaner for dishes, bathroom sinks and toilets. Instructions on the side of the bottle explain of how much concentrate to add to water depending on what you are cleaning. They also have a laundry detergent, again containing a bottle of Protective Blend. This is for newer HE washers, 1 tablespoon is used per load of laundry. We use this form of detergent in our house and are very pleased with the results.

In conclusion, safely store your oils ensuring purity and preventing breakdown, keep them in a cool, dry and dark place away from light and heat; a pantry, closet, or drawer is usually sufficient. Bathroom storage is discouraged due to the heat factor. Also maintain a tight seal or lid so that no air reaches them, or they will oxidize and evaporate. Theses oils are flammable so do not put them near an open flame.

To summarize please note the following DISCLAIMER: This chapter provides information on essential oils. It is not a substitute for medical advice. SAFETY PRECAUTIONS: Essential oils should not be used in the eyes, inside the ear canal or any mucous membranes. If redness or irritation occurs, apply a carrier oil to the affected area - water will not dilute essential oils. Citrus oils and blends containing them can increase sun sensitivity: allow at least 12 hours between application and exposing skin to the sun.

5 Nutritional Supplements

When choosing nutritional supplements, I am very selective to say the least. There are far too many products on the market that do not add up to the hype. First is the problem of cheap additives or excipients, fillers manufacturers use to keep the cost down. The problem then becomes one of quality. The human body prefers only natural ingredients; it accepts the synthetic ingredients by a subterfuge or a slight of hand. That means most supplement companies include a tiny portion of the natural ingredient along with mostly synthetic ingredients void of any nutritional benefits to make the body accept it. Aside from the fact that most excipients are void of any nutritional benefit, they are full of toxic chemicals that our bodies must process and excrete along with all of the other toxins in the SAD and environment which we are continuously exposed to.

We must look for excipients on the label for any vitamins we are considering. Excipients are binders, cheap fillers, and "glues" that have the capacity to damage the cell's DNA, which is in fact what all of the nutritional supplements are supposed to support! Some examples are: Magnesium Stearate - a cheap lubricating agent, Microcrystalline cellulose - a cheap filler, Silicon dioxide - a cheap flowing agent which is really sand, Triethyl citrate - a plasticizer, Titanium dioxide - used for coloring and toxic to the liver and Natural flavors - another name for monosodium glutamate which is a neurotoxin, Methyl paraben - a benzoate family member which is a known carcinogen and talcum powder - a common excipient rarely listed on product labels but a suspected carcinogen. Other questionable but common tableting and encapsulating agents include: D&C red #33,

Propylparaben, Hydroxyprpyl methylcellulose, Hydroxyprpyl cellulose, Polyethylene glycol, Red ferric oxide-orange shade, Methyl p-hydroxybenzoate, Propyl p-hydroxybenzoate, Sodium acetate, Methylparaben, Sodium metabisulfate and Eudragit. **Keep in mind that you never want to take a supplement in tablet form because it is compressed with tons of force becoming almost indigestible. This, coupled with the excipients I mentioned make tablets something to avoid.**

Currently, in my practice, I mainly use only a few brands of supplements and nutritional products. Of course this is always subject to change when newer, and more effective products are available.

It doesn't matter, which nutritional support you use, whether it is essential oils, supplements or both. We must all keep in mind that the intention is **ALWAYS focused on the BIG FOUR KEYS TO HEALTH: 1). DECREASING INFLAMMATION 2). OPTIMIZING DETOXIFICATION ABILITY 3). SUPPORTING THE IMMUNE SYSTEM 4). REJUVINATION/HEALING SUPPORT.**

In an attempt to decrease inflammation, we must enable the body to achieve an optimum pH, which is a reflection of the mineral content in the body. This is of utmost importance for good health. To determine the pH level, a person will test their first morning urine with a test strip any time after 5 am. This should be done daily for two weeks then averaged. This range should be between 6.4-7.4; it is preferable for the lower range to be closer to 7. Most Americans in this country have a pH between 5 - 6.2. due to the S.A.D. and that fact that the growing soil's mineral content is only 14% of what it was in 1934. In this case the body is leaching calcium from the bones to buffer this acidic pH in order to maintain balance. Makes you wonder about osteoporosis causes? When the body is finished with this calcium it leached from the bones, it must redeposit it usually between 5 - 7 a.m. often in the ears and eyes as calcium deposits; some tinnitus could actually be caused by this. The first nutritional product I recommend is from Immunologic: Its purpose is to achieve and keep an optimum pH. There are two products needed for this, one **pH Salts** and the other **Ionic Mineral Drops**. The salts contain calcium, magnesium, potassium, and sodium and the drops contain magnesium and 72 other minerals. I have tried products from other companies and found this is the only effective product to raise and maintain proper pH.

I must digress to talk briefly about one more product from Immunologic that I use: **Aloe Ferrox Whole Leaf.** The website describes it: "Aloe

Ferrox Whole Leaf contains both the aloin rich, raw bitter sap and the dried leaf for its polysaccharides, glyconutrients, chlorophyll, fiber, vitamins, minerals, amino acids, and fatty acids. Aloe Ferrox is a REMARKABLE constipation remedy while supporting normal bile flow for detoxification of liver and gallbladder and purification of blood. Indigenous to the Cape in South Africa, Aloe Ferrox is commonly used for immune support and bowel detoxification." In talking with the immunologic owner, Clive Buirski, he related the case of woman, constipated for thirty years, developed regular bowel movements after using this product. I also have had great success with constipated patients - most of them also hypothyroid.

The next product to decrease inflammation is from a company known as Premier Research Labs (PRL) founded by Dr. Robert Marshall, a PhD biochemist who actually cured himself of tryptophan poisoning twice using sound nutritional and whole nutrients after conventional medicine had no answer for him. PRL's mission is, "To empower every person to access their own limitless healing potential through the use of quantum resonance nutraceutical formulations, spectacular detoxification techniques and premier quality therapeutic strategies…." Interestingly, Clive Buirski worked for Dr. Marshall for many years before forming his own nutritional company, and they share much of the same philosophy. I cannot sufficiently praise the quality of their products. The PRL supplement line is extensive. In addition they offer a method of muscle testing, QRA or quantum research analysis that I have been trained in, as a means to identify what nutrients to prescribe. With QRA, there are acupuncture points which correspond to certain organs. When the acupuncture point is off – tests weak, the nutritional support is indicated. Thus, this is also an energy technique based on research from Dr. Fritz Popp, whose work I will discuss in the next chapter.

When attempting to manage inflammation in the body we have to address the subject of hormones. For overall hormone support we look to two supplements: **Deltanol** and **Tumeric**. Deltanol is the complete vitamin E consisting of four tocotrienols and not just the four tocopherols that most synthetic vitamin E supplements have. Tumeric, grown by Ayruvedic botanical growers, is imported from India. Dr. Marshall contends that "The hormone balance of body is a complex symphony of different regulating compounds, "which are, "The internal messengers that are necessary to control and regulate the body's processes." The organs in need of support here are the H/P/A axis (hypothalamic pituitary adrenals), thyroid, and reproductive glands. PRL has certain protocols consisting of two to three supplements to support the area needed. For example, for adrenal support there is **Adaptogen R3** and **Adrenoven**. Adaptogen consists of rare herbs such exotic herbs as Indian Soma Latha, Siberian Rhaponticum, Himalayan Rhodiola Rosea, Rhodiola Crenulata, Chinese Fo Ti Teng, European Opuntia and more. For thyroid support there is **Xenostat** and **ThyroVen**. Xenostat is full of naturally occurring iodine which enhances thyroid support. There is controversy over whether to give a person with an autoimmune thyroid condition any iodine because it will "add fuel to the fire." Most thyroid conditions, 90% in fact, are auto-immune in which the body attacks the thyroid, a condition known as Hashimotos, named after the Japanese doctor who discovered it. Opponents will argue that iodine will just create more TPO (thyroid peroxidase antibodies) which indicate an auto-immune flare-up. However, as Dr. Marshall has stated many times, Xenostat is a natural source of iodine, unlike the synthetic "garbage" iodine found in most of the other supplements, and will not aggravate a person with Hashimotos but will rather importantly support them.

For the reproductive organs and the hormones associated with them such as estrogen, progesterone and testosterone, PRL suggests the same supplement used for adrenal support that I just mentioned: Adaptogen-R3. There are also **Estro Flavone** and **Fem Balance-FX** for woman and **UltraPollen** and **Premier Testosterone** for men.

The second key to health is detoxification. Here I must refer to the initial chapter on toxic soup. Our exposure and bio-accumulation of toxic agents such as heavy metals, xenobiotics, pesticides and industrial chemicals warrants the body's periodic cleansing through detoxification; like the immune support - the third key major area of concern. Detoxification is a very broad topic and there are many PRL supplements for support. The liver is the main player needing support for detoxification, but before the liver can process food, we must address the stomach and small intestines. Ingested food needs sufficient HCL or hydrochloric acid to be secreted in order to be partially digested when it gets to the small intestine; otherwise it just sits there and putrefies, one of the problems with taking antacids. Thus to ensure there is proper stomach acid, PRL has the **HCL Detox kit** comprised of **HCL** and **HCL activator**. There is also PRL's **Digest** supplement taken before the detox kit to ensure proper digestive enzymes are present. The SAD and highly cooked foods deplete these enzymes; most Americans are deficient in them. Importantly, these digestive enzymes are also anti-inflammatory and help the HCL work better. The HCL is also the first line of defense for any bugs or bacteria eaten, killing them before they become problematic. The HCL activator is for the cells' re-methylation For the liver, there is **Max B ND**, and **Liver ND**. Because the kidneys play

Wellness in a Toxic World

a crucial role filtering 2000 liters of blood per day cleansing it, **RenaVen** is the main support for them helping to regulate mineral balance in the body.

The next category in the big four, the third key to health, is supporting immune function. This is such a broad topic, and there are so many supplements to support it that it could be the topic of an entire book.
First and foremost we need to protect against infections: yeast, fungi, viruses and bacteria. While addressing the other keys to health, the immune system is automatically addressed. Eighty percent of the immune system is located within our gut. With proper diet and digestion, the body is able to eliminate toxins and "guard the border" of the intestines effectively. Sometimes, however, an undigested piece of food known as "biofilm" is formed: 12-14 mm in size and too big for the macrophages or body's defense cells to enter. Infections know this and like to set up house in biofilms. PRL's answer to this is a supplement called **Allicidin. Another infection prevalent today with all of the sushi consumed are parasites. PRL has two key supplements for this, <u>Parastat</u> and <u>Paratosin</u>.**

Rejuvenation support is the fourth key to health. This is also a very broad subject and does involve numerous supplements including many of the ones already mentioned. I will only mention a few offered by PRL. **Premier Greens** contains a blend of Power Grass Plus Power Greens Blends air dried at low temperatures. **Lean Body Whey** has broad range antioxidant properties with a 5.000 ORAC (oxidative radical absorbance capacity). **Neuro-ND** contains resveratrol, the stabilizer for of DHLA (dihydrolipoic acid) and capable of quenching free radicals for superior anti-aging support.

PRL also has three products which meet a broad spectrum of fundamental nutritional needs and three of the four above key health factors including immune, hormone, whole body detoxification and rejuvenation support: **Ginseng FX -** known as the "king of all herbs," **Aloe Detox,** and **Medi-Clay FX -** a rare and believed to be the only known bentonite sourced from the site of an ancient underwater volcanic eruption that has been flushed with fresh water for millions of years.

For those beginning to investigate nutritional supplements or even using some synthetic multivitamin, now aware of their false claims and dangerous ingredients, PRL offers a "Getting started kit" consisting of a **Daily One** supplement and **Digest.** The Premier Daily one is an all in one daily formula for the whole family, a once living phytonutrient formula unlike the synthetic one – a - day vitamins flooding the market for over fifty years which are now even in "gummy bear" form loaded with sugar.

Like with the essential oils, many PRL supplements can be used to support many different conditions. That is the beauty of natural supplements; you can try different ones for better results without the harmful side effects of drugs if properly used.

In addition to their essential oils, dōTERRA has also formulated their own line of nutritional supplements based on them. These supplements contain only natural non-synthetic and pure ingredients. I want to discuss their flagship product known as the "Lifelong Vitality Pack." This consists of Cellular Vitality Complex, Essential Oil Omega Complex or Vegan EO Omega Complex, Food Nutrient Complex, and Energy and Stamina Complex providing a rich source of antioxidants.

Cellular Vitality Complex support contains proanthocyanidins from grape seeds, Baicalin from scutellaria root, Quercetin from Japanese Pagoda tree, Boswellic acids form Boswellia serrata, Resveratrol from Polygonum cuspidatum, Ellagic acid from pomegranate fruit extract, and Curcumin from Tumeric root. This blend of powerful polyphenols (compounds found in plants, fruits or vegetables that neutralize the damaging effects of free radicals) protect the cell's DNA, mitochondria and other vital cell structures. Along with the polyphenols, it contains a blend of essential fatty acids and therapeutic grade essential oils which all have clinically demonstrated the ability to support the cells' healthy oxidative stress response. To support the mitochondria or powerhouse of the cell for energy production, other co-factors in Cellular Vitality Complex ingredients include: Acetyl Carnitine which acts as a bus to transport fatty acids into the mitochondria, Alpha lipoic acid supporting this energy production, Coenzyme Q10 also supporting energy production and especially cardiovascular health. There are also other vitamins and minerals, co-factors needed to support the energy production and thus cell growth.

The next supplement included in the lifelong vitality program is either Essential Oil Omega Complex or Vegan EO Omega Complex. These two provide ultra-pure essential fatty acids and fat soluble vitamins to support healthy joints, the cardiovascular system, immune system, and brain health. The Essential Oil Omega Complex version uses a blend of marine and land based sourced essential fatty acids while the vegan version sources the blend of essential fatty acids from plant and algae based sources. There are countless numbers of toxins and contaminants in fish, squid, krill etc.; these forms of marine life eat the algae, which is the source of the essential fatty acids. I agree with the PRL position that it makes more sense to get rid of the middleman, the fish so to speak, and just take the plant sources. You might research this and come to your own a conclusion. Also included in either of these Essential Oil Omega Complexes is an antioxidant blend consisting of pure astaxanthin from microalgae and vitamin E, lutein, zeaxanthin, lycopene, and alpha/beta carotene. Finally, they both contain a blend of essential oils consisting of Clove, Frankincense, Thyme, Cumin, Wild Orange, Peppermint, Ginger, Caraway, and German Chamomile. Aside from their antioxidant function, this blend of essential oils functions to preserve and protect the marine essential fatty acids of the non - vegan Essential Oil Omega Complex from oxidation and rancidity - an inherent side effect with marine based essential fatty sources.

The third component of the lifelong vitality program is Food Nutrient Complex. This is a combination of essential vitamins and bio-available minerals to support energy production and immune function. Included is vitamins A, B complex, vitamin C, D and E. The minerals included are calcium, magnesium, copper, zinc, iron, selenium, manganese and chromium. A blend of trace minerals are also included for cellular metabolism. The body needs bio-available minerals in order to absorb vitamins. Whenever the word "essential" precedes vitamins or fatty acids it refers to those vitamin or acids which the body cannot manufacture on its own; they must be obtained from our diet. **However, it is common knowledge now that since the industrial revolution and the birth of GMO conglomerate Mont Santo, any nutrition is being grown out of our inferior foods due to current farming methods, pesticides and processing**. Our diet has changed but our genes, dependent on certain specific nutrients, are not receiving them. To remedy this, many unscrupulous supplement jam pack their vitamin formulas with everything they can. As, I said before and I am sure I will say it again, THE BODY DOES NOT RECOGNIZE SYNTHETIC SUBSTANCES. Most supplements on the retail market today contain only a small amount of a natural compound and are mostly synthetic which not only lacks any nutritional value but produces toxic effects as well.

Let me give some examples of the flagrant practice of selling mega doses of vitamins. Multivitamins began with the basic one a day vitamin based on the RDA (recommended daily allowance) between the years 1940-1950; the vitamins contained synthetic ingredients. During the 1980-1990s the vitamin companies began recklessly forming comprehensive - high dose multivitamins; their philosophy was that more must be better. Let's look at some specifics on the their ingredient list and compare it to the RDA's. The multivitamins were analyzed for individual vitamin and mineral content. Like the average American diet, one of the most common original multivitamins showed discrepancies in the quantities of optimum micronutrient with the RDA. For example, Vitamin A, a fat soluble vitamin which can build up in our system was at 150% of RDA whereas Vitamin C, D, and E were around 50%, 25%, and 50% respectfully. Folate, iron, iodine and manganese were over the 100% RDA with manganese being closer to 250% of the RDA! There were no fatty acids in this multivitamin. Let's fast forward to a more recent high end multivitamin. Vitamin A was at 60% RDA and there were no essential fatty acids. Vitamins D, K, iron, calcium and zinc were within 100% of RDA. Iodine,, copper and selenium and manganese are much higher than the 100% RDA at 150%, 200%, 250%, 350% RDA respectively. Everything else was way over the daily RDA - some even **off the chart or over 400% of the RDA?** This list includes: Vitamin C, E, B1, B2, B5, B6, B7, B9, B12, and chromium. Vitamin E is fat soluble and can build up to toxic levels in the body. Now it is true that since B vitamins are water soluble, they do not build up in our systems and must be replenished daily. However, the quality of most of the B vitamins for sale, including the ones in this comparison, are of inferior quality. That means they contain, not only 4 times the recommended safe, optimum limit, but also have the inferior ingredients and excipients bombarding the body which must deal with them.. If we now compare the Lifelong Vitality Pack supplements to the previous two generation of multivitamins we find that the longevity vitality product has all of the same nutrients falling within 100% of the RDA. To have the right quantity and quality without toxins is an incredible feat for a nutritional supplement. DōTERRA accomplishes this with their Lifelong Vitality Pack. I already discussed essential oils as support for the detoxification program; it also includes supplements. Now I want to discuss the supplements involved. To combat the toxicity of the SAD, which sabotages our digestive system and compromises the gut's immune system, dōTERRA has come up with a 30 day cleanse they recommend for people to do periodically.

The first supplement from dōTERRA for the 30 day cleanse is **GI Cleansing Formula**. Along with the proprietary blend of certified pure therapeutic grade essential oils, it also contains caprylic acid, a naturally derived fatty acid from coconut oil proven for over 40 years to support the balance of gut microbes by creating an unhealthy environment for potential threats interfering with normal digestion. This GI Cleansing Formula has been formulated to be used for 10 days as a preparatory phase before using the second supplement of the cleanse, **Probiotic Defense Formula.**

The Probiotic Defense Formula delivers 6 billion CFUs active probiotic cultures along with soluble fructo-oligosaccharides which actually encourage friendly bacterial growth. The capsule is unique in that it's double layered, providing a short chain pre-biotic fructo oligosaccharide in the outer portion and a time released active pro-biotic in the inner one. There are three proprietary strains of Lactobacillus promoting colonization and function of microflora higher in the intestinal tract and three strains of Bifidobacterium for healthy digestion and immune function of the lower intestine. This supplement is to be taken on the eleventh day - after the GI Cleansing Formula supplementation for 10 days are over and also must to be taken for ten days. After taking taking these two supplements for a total of 20 days, you simply skip the next 10. It is then recommended to take a product called **Digestive Enzyme Complex,** a proprietary blend of whole food digestive enzymes for the next 30 days. Due to the SAD loaded with processed foods, coupled with the lack of raw whole foods in the diet, digestive enzymes are overworked in the bodies like a worker pulling double shifts every day. Also, as we age, the production of digestive enzymes lessens. Digestive Enzyme Complex provides enzymatic support enhancing cellular metabolism resulting in healthier digestion. Finally, the fourth and last supplement recommended in the cleanse is **Detoxification Complex.** This product supports the excretory organs such as the skin, liver, kidneys, colon and lungs with a proprietary blend of whole food extracts specifically targeting the cleansing and filtering properties of these organs. This is taken along with Digestive Enzyme Complex for the next 30 days. It is recommended to do this cleanse about 2-3 times in succession to really clean out and rebuild the normal flora.

Another company whose products I use is Neurobiologix, founded by neurologist, Dr. Kendall Stewart. These products are for those discovered by genetic testing, to have methylation problem discussed in an earlier chapter. Although very complicated, genetic testing provides a deeper level or layer of investigation we sometimes when use when other treatments have been ineffective.

I must stress the crucial breakthrough of the 2003 completed **Human Genome Project study that discovered a gene, the methylenetetrahydrofolate reductase or MTHFR, is defective in many people - <u>especially those suffering from chronic health conditions.</u>**

Methylation of cells is such an important subject that it bares repeating some of my information. We need methyl groups for cell replication at the cells' DNA level. A methyl group is a carbon with three hydrogens (CH3) and is part of an acetyl group (COCH3). If there are not sufficient methyl groups for the proper methylation of cells to occur, then bad genes are turned on and protective genes are turned off, resulting in a chronic illness. Let me give some examples of methylation's necessary, multiple functions:

DNA/RNA synthesis (turn on/off genes), manufacturing brain neurotransmitters such as dopamine and serotonin, breakdown of hormones such as estrogen and testosterone, creation of natural killer and T immune cells, to create myelin coating on nerves, detoxification and the production of energy. Now if methylation does not occur when needed, here is what could result: cancer, diabetes, neurological disorders such as Parkinson's, Multiple Sclerosis, Alzheimer's, migraines, dementia, peripheral neuropathy, and hormonal issues such as PMS, ovarian cysts, fibroids, poly cystic ovary syndrome in women and low testosterone in men.

Some of the other nutritional products that I use successfully, from Neurobiologix, depend on the patient's genetic mutations found from genetic testing. Neuro-immune stabilizer is a cream promoting and enhancing methylation in order to assist in mood improvement, hormone regulation, sleep patterns and mental focus and concentration, to name a few. The advantage to using cream is its immediate absorption by skin, bypassing any malabsorption problems in the gastrointestinal tract which often arise. Calming cream is another product indicated when a neurotransmitter SNP biomarker on the genetic test is found. This cream promotes relaxation and assists with sleep disturbances and mood issues. Glutathione Plus can be indicated when a detox biomarker SNP is found on genetic testing and can be used in cases of heavy metal toxicity, Autism spectrum issues, chemotherapy toxicity, and chronic fatigue syndrome. Although some foods and many dietary supplements contain Glutathione, research has shown that it is not absorbed well when taken orally; topical Glutathione has been shown to be much more absorbable and effective. When an immune biomarker comes up on the genetic testing, a product called Mitochondria Restore is often indicated and assists with fatigue, growth delay, delayed healing, seizures and learning disabilities by significantly restoring the mitochondria's (powerhouse of the cell) ability to produce ATP. **I must add that some of these Neurobiologix products contain fillers such as sand and microcrystalline cellulose. I use them because I have found no other product yet as effective for methylation problems.**

Wellness in a Toxic World

6 Energy Medicine

My first introduction to energy medicine was the book, *Vibrational Medicine* by Richard Gerber MD. The concept that we are all vibrating at extremely fast frequencies enabling our being seen, is fascinating. Energy medicine is based on the conclusion that human beings are composed of a series of interacting multidimensional subtle energy systems. Thus, in a real sense, ***vibrational/energy medicine is Einsteinian medicine since his equation provides the key insight towards understanding that energy and matter are one in the same.*** When these energy systems get out of synch, pathological symptoms may result on the physical, mental, and spiritual planes. **(30)** In other words, when any human organism's system is weakened, and/or unbalanced, it will oscillate at a different frequency. Energy medicine maintains that these imbalances can be rectified by rebalancing the subtle energies with the right vibrational frequency.

Obviously this is a hard pill to swallow for Western medicine. That there is an "etheric" component to our physical being does not sit well with most pragmatic thinking. The **Etheric** Body gives vitality, health, life and organization to the Physical Body. It attunes our consciousness to the principle of energy. We are more than just flesh and bones, cells and proteins; we are beings composed of the stuff of the universe or frozen light composed of many different frequencies - a bioplasma, one concept of a universal energy in which all objects are interconnected with the energy flowing between them; the crux of energy medicine.

In this chapter, I will discuss energy medicine broadly: the differences between orthodox and alternative medicine, or the Newtonian versus Einsteinian model, and then will give examples of commonly known energy techniques as well as those we incorporate in this office.

Traditional western, not eastern, orthodox medicine has always depended solely on drugs and surgery; this is based on the Newtonian model of reality in which psychological and physiological behavior is dependent on the structure of the brain and body. This model views the body like an intricate clock. Traditional medicine can replace a heart with a mechanical replacement and could even mimic the job of the kidneys with a dialysis machine, but sadly to this day the knowledge to reverse or even prevent many disease still evades them. Drug therapy, like surgery, targets a certain tissue in hopes of correcting the problem without the use of a scalpel. Today there have been strides in molecular biology, however, enabling better diagnosis and treatment of human illness but this Newtonian mechanistic approach only looks at the body's hardware; organs, enzymes and cells void of the "life force" needed to breathe life to these tissues, and is therefore only a partial truth of the body's reality. Thus, unlike a machine, human beings are much more than a sum of their physical parts due to this synergism. The human body is constantly renewing its vehicle of expression - the cells. **(31)** <u>Applied to the universe, the Newtonian model purports that it is composed of separate atoms with protons and electrons.</u>

This life force or energy, is shunned by the medical profession because of the lack of an acceptable scientific model explaining its existence. The Newtonian Model wanted to remove divine explanations from "the mystical forces that move humans through life, and just as mysteriously, through sickness and death." Although crucial to furthering mechanical advancements during the industrial revolution, the Newtonian model had many shortcomings such as the failure to explain the behavior of electricity and magnetism, therefore new scientific models were needed. The problem was, however, the scientific community in charge of medical research was still working from a Newtonian model: a cellular mechanism devoid of vital tissue animating energies. As stated earlier, since the mid twentieth and half of this century, great scientific advancements have led to a greater understanding of molecular interaction with physical matter but bioenergetics fields influencing cellular patterns, growth and physical
expression were not investigated. Contrary to this Newtonian mechanistic model, we have those scientists who try to understand the functioning of the human body based on the view of matter as energy. Hence, we have the Einsteinian model: humans are beings of energy. By ascribing to this belief system, we not only can have a unique perspective on the cause of many diseases, but we can many insights on the inner workings of nature and the

secrets of the universe as well.

Understanding Einstein's model requires an understanding of laser light which is coherent and extremely orderly and focused, like military cadets marching in formation. Everyone has heard of using surgical lasers for eye lens correction, but lasers can also be used to illuminate different patterns. Holograms are a special picture created from three dimensional energy interference patterns. An example of interference patterns in nature is when two stones are dropped simultaneously in a calm pool of water; when the two groups of circular waves meet they interact forming an interference pattern. Holigraphically, this means that if you cut away a small piece of the holographic film, an entire intact and three dimensional image of the photographed image results. **(32)** The study of Holograms has led to a more in-depth study and understanding of Einsteinian physics which would never have occurred using the simple deductive reasoning and logic of the Newtonian model. Now in order to apply the holographic principles to the human body we just look at the cells. Remember from genetics that every cell in the human body contains a copy of the body's DNA or blueprint containing enough information to make an entire new body. This parallels the holograph's principle that every piece contains the information of the whole. Holograms really give us a new, unique model which can aid science in understanding not only energetic patterns of human beings but the structure of the universe. <u>Thus, Einstein's theories of Quantum physics proved that the Universe is composed of particle waves that interact with each other despite the distance in space between them and they are void of any time constraint: part of the universal intelligence</u>. Modern orthodox medicine's explanation of cell differentiation can be explained using molecular biology and DNA. However, to put it simply, what it cannot explain is how the cells know where to go and how to line up in a certain spatial relationship, if you will. This is the function of the physical body; a holographic "etheric body" which carries the information for a spatial template and for cellular repair in case there is damage, for example, to the developing fetus. Proof of this etheric body was the main agenda for Harold Burr in the 1940s, a scientist from Yale University, using salamanders, he studied the shape of the electric fields surrounding them. While mapping these electrical fields in salamander embryos, he discovered that the electrical axis originated in the unfertilized egg, a contradiction to the conventional biological and genetic theory of his day. Burr injected a dark indelible ink into salamander eggs using a micropipette technique and discovered that it always became incorporated into the brain and spinal cord of the developing fetus. He also experimented with seedlings and found that the electrical field surrounding them was not the shape of the original seed but instead the shape of the adult plant suggesting a growth template is followed. This data also suggested that this growth template was generated by the organism's individual magnetic field. **(33)** Giving more credence to the bioenergetics growth fields was the research by a Russian named Seyon Kirlian who pioneered electrography or Kirlian photography in the early 1940s, about the same time Burr's research was conducted.

This is a technique in which living objects are photographed in the presence of a high frequency, high voltage, and low amperage electric field. Both Burr and Kirlian's experiments were capable of measuring changes in the energy fields of living systems; the former used a skin voltmeter and the latter visual electrical measurements. Both men also found that diseases such as cancer caused significant changes in the electromagnetic fields of living organisms. Kirlian recorded these changes as corona discharge images to confirm disease associated energy fields. **(34)**

MRI (magnetic resonance imaging) has been incredible in evaluating the physical and biochemical components of the human cellular framework by evaluating the distribution of molecular structure and biochemical function. Yet, what is missing is an imaging system allowing doctors to evaluate this energetic component; conventional medicine does not have sufficiently sophisticated equipment to allow evaluation of the energetic component. The etheric structure has a frequency spectrum much higher than that of physical matter measured by MRI. Subatomic particles of physical matter such as electrons can trace delicate outlines associated with the body of a leaf when stimulated with etheric high frequencies. Some of the readers may have heard of "the phantom leaf effect" done with Kirlian photography methods. Thus, the energies used in Kirlian are not the identical frequency of the etheric body consisting of lower octaves of the higher vibrational energies. This is the primary difference between MRI and an EMR (electromagnetic resonance) imaging system such as Kirlian photography. In other words, a leaf is on the surface and then removed. A picture is taken and the outline of the leaf remains, its energetic signature. In the future, a CAT Scan like imaging system may be developed taking cross sectional slices which could then be added together to create a 3 dimensional picture of the etheric body. This could identify problems with the etheric body before they manifest in the physical body as cellular changes. For now, however, *the phantom leaf effect remains as the best candidate for a photograph of the etheric body of a living organism.*

Perhaps the biggest proof that the bioenergetics field around the body is not completely separated from the physical body is exemplified by the ancient Chinese practice of acupuncture. There are specific channels of energy exchange allowing the flow of energetic information to move between the body systems. *This form of healing has been around for over 3000 years but was not acknowledged by western medicine until recently*. In Acupuncture theory, acupuncture points run alongside unseen meridians or information pathways running deeply throughout the tissues at certain locations of the body. The Chinese believe that there are 12 pairs of meridians connected to specific organ systems and that Chi is the energy passed along theses invisible pathways. When blocked or imbalanced, dysfunction of that organ system will result. Energy polarity is another key concept of Chinese philosophy expressed by "yin" and "yang." Yin is viewed as the female particle; passive, destructive, associated with the moon, darkness and death. Yang on the other hand is the male principle: active, generative, associated with sun, light, and the creative principle of life. Reflecting an energetic oscillation between polar opposites, both of these are needed to maintain balance in the universe in all aspects of all life cycles. In order to have birth, death must also occur. I am not trained in acupuncture, therefore, do not use it in my office but feel that it has many merits and does seem to be the only "energy medicine" technique accepted by the conventional medical profession and it is covered by many insurance policies.

Another very well-known energy technique, homeopathy, is unfortunately not as accepted as acupuncture by the conventional medical profession. I am not a homeopath and do not use traditional homeopathy in my office. However, since homeopathy is very well known to those in "alternative medicine" and has philosophical appeal separating it from traditional orthodox medicine, I will explain it. Interestingly, it has been used by Queen Elizabeth ll and the royal family with success for many years and was praised in 2012 in a Swiss article extolling its success. Unfortunately, in 2014 Australia released a negative article arguing that, "it does not work, and is not better than a placebo." Perhaps it was working too well that the medical profession had to defame it; I see it as an another attempt to discredit a non-conventional medical treatment. Homeopathy has been around for the past 250 years; it must have done something right to survive this long?

A German physician, Samuel Hahnemann is credited with being the discoverer of Homeopathy following his disillusionment with the traditional medical approaches of his day. He studied Greek medical principles available in German folk medicine called "like cures like" and developed a system of healing based on this. For instance, if a healthy person took a certain homeopathic remedy for a sore throat, for example, the remedy would give the healthy person a sore throat, but would cure the sick patient having a sore throat. This was later formalized into a concept known as "law of similars." Hahnemann reasoned that a remedy created an artificial illness giving the same symptomatic picture as the disease and then stimulate the body's immune system to fight it. This follows a principle known as VIS Medicatrix Naturae, or if translated, "the healing powers of nature." In modern day homeopathy these symptoms a remedy induces are known as the homeopathic "drug picture." An important difference between Homeopathy and conventional medical thinking is the emphasis placed on the mental and emotional symptoms as opposed to simply physical symptoms; the medical profession placed the greatest weight with the latter and homeopathy on the former. During Hahnemann's research, he discovered *diluting the remedy made it stronger and more effective. and* referred to this as "potentization." Some of his remedies were so diluted that there were no molecules of the original herb remained. Obviously, this was a huge contradiction to the accepted medical principles of the times dealing with dose related drugs. CONVENTIONAL DOCTORS BELIEVE THAT IN ORDER FOR ADMINISTERED DRUGS TO HAVE THERAPUTIC EFFECTS UPON THE BODY'S CELLULAR RECEPTORS, THEY MUST BE GIVEN IN DOSAGES HIGH ENOUGH TO BE MEASURED WITH A BLOOD TEST. Many drug minded people cannot accept this point: Zero molecules of an original substance have significant physical and psychological effects on the body.

It's necessary to understand that the energetic portion of the remedy is the source of the strength not the actual substance. The Newtonian model fails to explain this, therefore, we must turn to the Einsteinian model or subtle energy model for the reasons of the healing properties of such dilute molecular solutions.

Let me briefly explain how a homeopathic solution is made. After a plant is soaked in alcohol, a drop of this tincture is taken and mixed with either 10 or 100 parts water. For example, there can be a 1:10 dilution and a 1:100 dilution which is then shaken forcefully, in a process known as succussion. One drop of water taken from this solution is added to 10 or 100 parts water depending on the strength of solution needed, always maintaining the same ratio. It is both succussed and diluted again and continually until the desired dilution is achieved in a technique known as "potentization." The number of atoms in a mole is roughly 6×10^{23rd} so that by the 12th dilution of a $10x$ 24th potency, it is unlikely that even a single atom of the original substance is left! **(35)** These potencies can get very high; in the UK, for example, doctors use the centesimal scale in which you can have a 10 to the 6th power dilution and a 10 to the 30th. I mentioned earlier that homeopathy believes that there must be equal emphasis placed on the body's psychological and physical aspects. The former dilution mostly targets the body's physical tissues and the latter dilution targets the psychological aspects. **(36)**

Therefore, homeopathic remedies are subtle energy remedies containing the "vibrational signature" of the plant from which they came. **It is these vibrational signature frequencies which provide the healing benefits not the molecular properties of the substance**. Thus, if the chosen remedy matches the frequency of the patient's illness, there will be a resonant transfer of energy allowing the bioenergetic field of the patient to utilize this needed energy to remove toxins or microbes and achieve an improved level of health.

PRL supplements and dōTERRA essential oils are also categorized as energy medicine. They both target the energetic signature of the organ or tissue they are designed to resonate with. Each recognizes the bioenergetic field around the body and the photons of light each cell has and uses a method of analysis, in Dr. Marshall's words for, "precisely identifying the hierarchy of what is going on in the human body." PRL uses QRA (quantum reflex analysis) which is an analysis of the bio-energy field by muscle testing at various acupuncture points on the body corresponding with certain organs to determine the best nutritional supplement to turn on the weak or challenged acupuncture point. To decide which essential oils the body needs, we use a bio-feedback device known as the Zyto scan, which I discussed earlier in this book.

PRL also has a myriad of household products such as "The Trilliant Pyramid, "the "crowning glory" in vastu remediation made with a 52 degree slope like the pyramids of Giza. It is comprised of highly conductive metals offering outstanding repolarization of a house, for example, that combats the depolarization effect of the killing "energy" vectors in the average home improperly laid out. These pyramids also provide the most beneficial frequencies to date and work best when a house is grounded first.

When we look at how this energy flows through the body, we need to reference Ancient Indian yogic literature which describes special energy centers within our subtle body referred to as "chakras," a word derived from the Sanskrit word for "wheels" resembling whirling vortices of subtle energies emanating from the major nerve plexus branching forward from the spinal column. There are seven major chakras in the body correlating with both a major nerve plexus and an endocrine gland. They are located near the coccyx to the crown of the head, from lowest to highest. There are actually two different chakra systems, one born of the Eastern race and one born of the Western race. Some practitioners speculate a merger between the two would result in a new chakra system. For now, the main difference between the two systems is that Easterners and Westerners put different emphasis on certain chakras. Regardless, chakras translate high frequency energy between auric levels (auric levels correspond to chakras) and into a gland/hormone output which affects the entire body. Chakras have been metaphorically compared to flowers distributing their subtle energies into the body and they also bring about the development of different aspects of self-consciousness. Chakras differ from the meridians which have a physical counterpart in their meridian duct system. **(37)**

Applied kinesiology is a great example of an energetic test performed on the body. It is the study of the relationship between muscle strength and health. It was developed by a chiropractor, Dr. George Goodhart, in 1964 and was based on the theory that a body's dysfunction is accompanied by muscular weakness. A variety of methods including supplements to herbs, homeopathy etc., are used to treat the muscle weakness then a re-test follows seeking a strong muscle indicating resolution of the problem.

There are many types of Energy therapy along with the two major examples acupuncture and homeopathy. Another therapy is called healing touch, based on the transfer of energy through the laying on of hands. It was founded by an RN, Janet Mentgen, in 1989 whose incentive was to form a deeper connection between nurses and their patients.

Chinese therapy known as Qi Gong, unfortunately most often considered by many in the westerns to be a form of martial arts: this is really an ancient Chinese system of postures, exercise, breathing techniques, and meditations designed to enhance the body's Qi (pronounced Chi) or vital life force.

Polarity therapy, another form, measures the aura of bio-energetic field around our bodies. Metal rods, forked tree branches, and even pendulums of various types have historically been used for 4,000 years to prove the existence of the field according to archeologists. As practiced today, however, it may have originated in Germany during the 1400s when it was used to find ground metals; Vietnam soldiers used dowsing to locate weapons and tunnels. In addition to measuring auric fields, dowsing rods have also been used to find water, metals, gemstones, oil, and currents of the earth's among others. The basis of how this works lies in large changes in electrical conductivity. Einstein wrote, "The dowsing rod is a simple instrument which shows the reaction of the human nervous system to certain factors, which are unknown to us at this time." This begs the question of whether we have another sensory system we are not consciously aware of.?

The healing touch, or "Reiki," is yet another energy therapy. My wife Becky happens to be a certified Reiki practitioner and administers this therapy in our office. This Japanese technique aims at stress reduction, relaxation and the promotion of healing by transferring energy through the palms to heal and balance the bio-electric/aura field of the body. This therapy can be traced back thousands of years to the ancient cultures of India, Tibet, China, and Japan. It fell into obscurity, but was rediscovered in the middle 1800's by a Japanese theologian, Dr. Mikao. The word Reiki combines two words "Rei" and "Ki" which mean spiritual wisdom and life energy. This life energy is the same as Chinese "Chi" or "Prana" in Sanskrit. It is otherwise known as biofeild energy and constitutes the universal life energy. The life force animating all living things must flow freely, or there will be health consequences. The "Ki" in Reiki is a special kind of Ki guided by spiritual consciousness; it heals because it balances the life energy by flowing through the chakra, meridian, and nadis pathways nourishing the organs and tissues as well as flowing around our aura. Because it is guided by spiritual consciousness, Reiki can never do any harm. Both practitioner and client are in need of healing and thus receive benefit from a session: An increase in energy and feelings of love and well-being are the result.

I would be remiss if I did not discuss Royal Rife and the "True Rife machine." A gifted researcher who dedicated his life to the link between electromagnetic energy and cancer, invented a microscope that could magnify organisms up to thirty thousand times using a polarized light which would glow a particular color depending on the organism viewed. This extremely high magnification allowed the organism to be viewed alive, unlike the slides of dead, stained organisms others researched. He discovered that each organism resonated at its own frequency; he would then subject these live organisms to various frequencies using a device he invented known as the Rife beam ray that would inflict what Rife called the MOR or mortal oscillating frequency. Within moments of being hit with these frequencies, the bacteria stopped moving and died. He had tremendous success destroying bacteria in people afflicted with infectious disease, even chronic recurrent infections like bone infection Osteomyelitis in which the bacteria are resistant to antibiotics. Rife also believed that cancer was caused by a virus.

"Although Rife's work was strongly criticized by the conventional medical authorities of his day, many cancer research laboratories have since found evidence of viral DNA in certain human cancers." (38) In 1934, he was a member of an investigational cancer research study at the University of Southern California, where he used his Rife beam daily at three minute intervals on 16 terminally ill cancer patients. Miraculously, three months later, thirteen out of sixteen were pronounced, by the staff, cured. Furthermore, he had a 90% cure rate with all types of cancer. What happened to this great man's treatment is a travesty. Morris Fishbein, editor of the Journal of the American Medical Association tried to buy and take control of the rife technology, but Rife refused the offer. Because, Fishbein could not control the Rife beam use, he wanted to shut it down. Conveniently, a short time later, a laboratory built to study the Rife machine burned down? Interestingly, due to Fishbein's connection with high ranking medical officials, Rife was dragged through the California court systems resulting in the immediate nonuse declaration of any Rife machines. This great cancer treatment was never looked at further until the latter part of the twentieth century. Interestingly, Fishbein was later convicted of Racketeering charges. Today, people can purchase a Rife machine but must be cautious; there are many available knockoff models on the market. Many doctors on my forums rent these machines or have their cancer patients purchase them. For a proper treatment, the patient must be near this machine for a few hours per day and then should actually sleep with the light emitting frequency bulb.

To understand how these energy therapies work, we must look at the electromagnetic theory of healing, pioneered by Dr. William Tiller, a materials science professor at Stanford. During the nineties, he was trying to correlate current scientific models with the subtle energy theory. Dr. Richard Gerber actually coined the term for this work, the "Tiller-Einstein model of positive-negative space/time." He calls it this because the famous equation, $E=mc^2$ relates energy to matter - energy is inherent in matter. This is the abbreviated equation known as the "Einstein-Lorentz Transformation." It has a relativistic factor describing different parameters of measurement: Alteration of mass and time will vary depending on the velocity of the system. **(39) Einstein's equation signifies that there is a tremendous amount of potential stored energy within tiny particles of matter.** For example, a few teaspoons of uranium in atomic bomb will unleash devastating damage. **Einstein's energy theory has evolved over time and to many scientists has given us a more multidimensional view of the universe in which matter and energy are both interconvertible and interconnected**. This brings us to the subtle energy: If the equation applies to gross matter and energy, (the atomic bomb) does it also apply subtle matter and energy? To reach the dimensional aspects of matter., Einstein's $E=mc^2$, x it must be accelerated to the speed of light and beyond. Some people do not believe that it is possible to travel beyond the speed of light however, such pioneering mathematicians like Charles Muses consider the square root of -1 belonging to a category of numbers referred to as 'hypernumbers' that he believes are necessary to validate higher dimensional phenomena with equations to describe the subtle energies in living systems I have described thus far. **(40)**

I must repeat at this point that all matter whether physical or subtle energy, has frequency and matter with different frequencies that co-exist together, just as radio and TV. **(41)** Thus the etheric (subtle) and physical bodies co-exist and overlap being different frequencies. **Energy blockages or disturbances in the etheric body precede the physical or cellular manifestation of illness**. <u>We must address the body's bio-energetic field and balance it in order to balance the physical body</u>!

On the elliptical at the gym this morning, I saw a clip on a news channel from the movie "Back To the Future" in which Marty Mcfly was riding a hover board while being chased. The news showcased the real life hover board that Lexus is developing. It made me think how scientists apply the laws of physics to develop sophisticated weapons, medical equipment, social media devices, etc. Energy medicine also applies these same quantum physics principles to the human body.

"Everything is energy and that's all there is to it. Match the frequency of the reality you want and you cannot help but get that reality. It can be no other way. This is <u>not</u> philosophy. This is <u>physics</u>."
–Albert Einstein

7. Field Control Therapy (FCT)

Field control therapy is a form of energy medicine known as "causative homeopathy." Unlike the classic homeopathy I previously discussed, this focuses solely against the offending agents instead of the symptoms these agents cause. **(42)** Developed by a board certified cardiologist, Dr. Savely Yurkovsky in 1999, who was disenchanted with conventional medicine and their "dismal yield in the care of chronic diseases," so he explored the alternative medicine field. Dr. Yurkovsky was aware that the cellular fields were the primary source of health and disease, so he developed a revolutionary model combining theories of physics and biology which were established by his mentor, Professor Emeritus of Materials Science, William A. Tiller of Stanford University.

I must thank one of my colleagues from the "Johnson Group," a neurometabolic group of doctors from around the country who exchange valuable health information, for the following profound statement about FCT. "Field Control Therapy is a relatively new healthcare system that specifically addresses the illnesses of the 21st century. Modern lifestyle comes at a cost. Poor diet, increased exposure to radiation, environmental pollutants and toxic metals are creating a host of new health problems from chronic fatigue to immunodeficiency, autism and multiple sclerosis, to name a few. FCT identifies key toxins underlying illness and treats with 'causative homeopathy' to restore healthy cellular functioning."

Vibrational medicine is the basis of how FCT works. It has been known for decades that molecules vibrate, and that every atom of every molecule gives off certain frequencies, an essential physical characteristic of matter. Specific frequencies of molecules can be detected from billions of light years by radio telescopes. If we look around the physical world and realize that there are over one billion atoms in a grain of sand, it is difficult to understand how many atoms and frequencies we must deal with. An atom contains electrons, protons, neutrons, etc. of course, but these occupy only tiny specs inside the atom; the rest is mostly *empty space*. The human body contains about one hundred trillion cells; how well these cells interact determine your state of health. It is estimated that each cell undergoes close to 100,000 chemical reactions each second. This means that the tiny specs of the atoms of the cells interact at a rate that is almost beyond comprehension. Our ability to detoxify toxins, to heal, to regulate metabolism, the ability to sleep, the appearance of the skin and the ability to properly digest food, are determined by the effectiveness of this interaction. Because nutrition directly affects these specs it is imperative that they are healthy and can perform their function. **WORKING WITH THE SPECS IN THE CELLS IS <u>BIOCHEMISTRY</u>**.

But what about the space between the specs of the atom within the body's cells. Life depends on the signals exchanged between molecules. Think about what happens to cause physiological changes to occur. For example, what tells the body to increase blood pressure or make the heart beat faster, or to raise body temperature? The words "molecular signal" are used freely in biology; yet, the concept of the way the information is exchanged between the cell and its receptor to produce a physiological response to occur does not exist in mainstream biology. According to Dr. Yurkovsky, this truth based fact is simple and "does not require a collapse of the physical or chemical worlds." A German physicist, Dr. Fritz-Albert Popp, PhD in theoretical physics and a professor at Mainz University, has conducted extensive research confirming the existence of biophotons. These particles of light consist of a high order of light, otherwise known as a biological laser, showing a very stable intensity without the normal fluctuations normally observed in light. Dr. Popp states, "<u>Because of the high degree of coherence (high degree of order), the biological "laser" light is able to generate and keep order and also to transmit information in the organism.</u>" His experiments show that the living cells' DNA stores and releases photons creating "biophotonic emissions" that may hold the key to illness and health; thus biophotons participate in the regulation of a wide spectrum of biological and physiological functions. This phenomenon has been experimentally verified, in unicellular organisms by many governmental and university research laboratories. These separate cell cultures exhibit photon communication resulting in synchronization of their emission pattern in the tissues and organs of animals and humans, and in plants. **Interestingly, tumor cells were found to exhibit characteristic photon emission pattern different from normal cells.** These biophotons participate in the regulation of a wide spectrum of biochemical and physiological functions. Dr. Fritz Popp wrote 8 books and more than 150 scientific journal articles and studies addressing basic questions on theoretical physics, biology, complementary medicine and biophotons. **WORKING WITH THE SPACE BETWEEN THE CELLS IS <u>BIOPHYSICS</u>.**

Remember Dr. Harold Burr, from chapter six, who studied the electric field around a salamander. An orthopedic surgeon, Dr. Robert Becker, was fascinated with bio-electricity or electricity in living things. He was also a professor at the State University of New York. And like Dr. Burr, he experimented with salamanders in an attempt to discover what causes limb regeneration. He did extensive research on this topic and wrote *The Body Electric* and eventually developed a widely accepted technique for stimulating bone healing using electric stimulation. **Not known at the time, the electrical signals Dr. Becker was detecting in the bodies of both animals and humans, were part of the body's energy system!** He also published another book, *Cross Currents* in which he described a "data transmission and control system" located in cells, transmitting information by means of a DC (direct current.). Dr. Becker received a Nobel prize nomination for his work.

Dr. Yurkovsky did eight years of research in the early 1990s following a purely experimental approach and discovered that specific molecular signals could be transferred using an amplifier and electromagnetic coils. He recorded and replayed these signals on a computer soundcard in 1995. Over the course of several thousand experiments he led receptors to "believe" that they were in the presence of their favorite molecule simply by playing the molecule's recorded frequencies. The frequency spectrum range in which a molecular signal can be effectively represented is between 20-20,000 Hz - the same range as human hearing and music. Dr. Yurkovsky pointed out that "for thousands of years, humans have been relating sound frequencies to a biological mechanism: the emotions." Composers of background music for supermarkets and elevators are practicing neurophysiology without knowing it!. High pitched rapid sounds engender lightness of spirit; high pitched slow sounds, sweetness, sounds both deep and rapid awaken the fighting spirit, while deep, slow sounds invoke serious emotions, sadness, and mourning. These are fundamentally cerebral physicochemical phenomena, triggered by defined frequencies. We do nothing more than this when we transmit pre-recorded molecular activities to biological systems." A modern day example of using frequencies as a diagnostic means is an EKG machine which measures the frequency of the heart.

Let me reference the radio in relation to the human body. Radio stations have different frequencies just like body tissues and organs have their own unique frequencies. If you want a certain radio station you must plug in the exact frequency to get it or else static results. This also holds for the body's individual organ frequencies. If the thyroid gland, for example, normally resonates at 68 MHz but because of a bad diet and other environmental toxins, now is resonating at 55 MHz, the functioning of it will be less than optimal; analogous to radio static.

By now, we have established that the body has an electric field around it, the bioelectric field. Many people are not aware that the brain produces 30 watts of electricity - enough to light a light bulb. (For all the at- least- fifty-something crowd reading this, I just had the image of Uncle Fester with the light bulb in his mouth). The bio electric field around our bodies also contains a magnetic component making it an electromagnetic field. To demonstrate this to my patients, I use an energy stick. When we both touch one end of the stick with one hand and then touch each other with the other hand, the stick lights up because of the electromagnetic energy we are releasing completes the circuit. This is, of course, an invisible effect but nevertheless true. Think of looking at two common magnets; you can hold them apart and they are attracted to each other one way and then if you turn them over they repel each other. Can you see the actual force that does this? The earth also has this same magnetic field. Just think of the sailors several centuries ago navigating their ships with a compass. Extraordinarily, not only does the human body generate an electromagnetic field around it, but it can even be measured several feet away from the body!

The uniqueness about the body's "energy language" is that it is about 100 times more efficient than the chemistry language (specs in cells and all of the daily myriad reactions). In other words, when the cells communicate, the energy field is required to tell the biochemical mechanism what to do, not the other way around - this is a one way street because of the speed required; it could not be reversed. Consequently, if conventional medicine neglects to test and treat the bio electromagnetic field, they have only read one or two chapters of a book so to speak. This may be why I often see patients who feel out of sorts and have been told by their family doctor that there is nothing wrong with them; their blood work and other tests are normal? **These conventional practitioners are not reading all of the** chapters in the book.

Let's look at the many sources that interfere with this electromagnetic field's communication with the physical body. Remember the initial chapter, "A Toxic Soup" for these sources: heavy metal toxicities from amalgam fillings for example, yeast, pesticides such as Roundup, mold, fungus, bacteria, viruses, herbicides, parasites, over the counter and prescription medication residues, GMO foods, chemical laden hygiene products, fish farms, wireless internet, remote car start, cell phones, cell phone towers, computers, microwaves, the S.A.D., vaccinations etc.... The list goes on. Many of the increasingly prevalent chronic conditions most Americans suffer from, cancer, cardiovascular disease, and Alzheimer's can result from these sources. Why do you think this is? **WE LIVE IN A WORLD OF TOXICITY AND EMFs.** There is no escape from the toxic load. You can, however, drastically reduce your exposure to many of these toxic sources. These deterrents adversely affect the body's normal organ frequency ranges. Let's look at some deterrents and their interference with the body's bioenergy field.

Despite the ongoing controversy surrounding mercury's high toxicity to humans, it amazingly continues to be very popular in America.
In his book, *It's All In Your Head,* Dr. Hal Huggins describes how he developed a method of identifying those people sensitive to mercury in amalgam dental fillings. This study showed measurable changes in temperature, blood pressure, and pulse in those sensitive to mercury. Moreover, not only do amalgam fillings contain mercury, they also contain zinc, copper, silver and tin. Dr. Higgins found a whopping 90-96% of these patients were sensitive not only to mercury but also to copper and zinc, and 63-67% patients were sensitive to the sliver and tin metals.

Mercury is by far the most prevalent and insidious of the heavy metals. A phrase has been coined depicting this called "micro-mercurialsm" the way it builds up in our system over time. This metal is found mostly in farm raised fish, vaccinations in the thimerosal form, fluorescent lights and dental amalgams. Dr. Huggins's research has demonstrated that mercury attacks the body in five ways: neurological, cardiovascular, collagenous, immunological, and miscellaneous including chronic fatigue, brain fog, digestive problems and Crohn's disease. The ADA or American Dental Association, thirty years ago, declared that 5% of the population were sensitive to mercury found in amalgam fillings containing 50% mercury. Speaking at a convention, Dr. Huggins, reminding the ADA that 5% is an epidemic and would constitute 12.5 million Americans, the ADA immediately reduced that number to 1%. Guess what, the ADA never loses; the patient is the loser. **(44)**

It is not advisable for those with amalgam fillings to have them removed unless the procedure is done by a holistic dentist; there will be considerable mercury released that could adversely affect the patient and even cause an unsuspected chronic disease in the future. The holistic dentist will take precautions on removing the fillings and what should replace them. Go to the website, **www.toxicteeth.org,** for more information and holistic dentists. I live in Carlisle PA; there are three holistic dentists within an hour from me, all in PA - one in Hershey, one in Columbia and one in Halifax. They should be IAOMT accredited meaning they are trained and tested in biocompatible dentistry including current methods for safe removal of dental amalgams.

For those people who prefer to keep their amalgam fillings, fear not. Using FCT, I am actually able to treat the mercury toxicity in a safe way so that the fillings do not adversely affect your health.

The ubiquitous weed killer roundup, also known as Glyphosate, is very toxic, and labeled GMO (genetically modified). It has a half - life of 22 years. The powerhouse of the cell, the mitochondria, is greatly affected by this pesticide; anyone exposed to it produces less energy. Glyphosate kills the soil's good bacteria the same way the SAD kills the good bacteria in the gut, resulting in a corn stalk, for example, that does not fully decompose. When the farmer tills the soil, that stalk is worked back into it and the viscous cycle continues. Moreover, because the GMO corn affects the nervous systems of the cows who eat it, as you may have guessed this meat will also be used in food processing for pets and humans, a good example of the viscous cycle.

Man-made EMFs (electromagnetic fields), known as electrosmog, consist of frequencies of 50-60Hz and include the high voltage power lines coming into our houses and the appliances that run off that electricity. Some of the more common examples are: hair dryers, electric blankets, refrigerators, alarm clocks, televisions, computers, and compact fluorescent lights. Electric blankets, even when turned off, can penetrate up to 6 inches into the body, and some studies linked them to miscarriages. Alarm clocks have a harmful electric field up to 3 feet away and have been linked to brain tumors from chronic exposure. With chronic exposure, Compact fluorescent lights (CFL) emit ultraviolet radiation which can increase the chances of skin cancer. CFLs also generate a higher "electrosmog" field - more than the tube fluorescent lights and are closer to a person increasing their exposure since they are in a lamp. The third reason the CFLs are so harmful is that they contain mercury inside - one of the most toxic and lethal heavy metals and a serious constant threat if a bulb is broken or dropped. The WHO (World Health Organization) found in a recent study that CFL exposure precipitated a wide range of symptoms from skin problems and fatigue to heart palpitations and digestive problems. In 1996, the EPA (Environmental Protection Agency) found a correlation between harmful extremely low frequencies of 60 Hz and cancer. The White House and Air Force did not wish to "alarm" the public and "apparently tried to suppress these findings." The EPA also had studies showing a consistent pattern of response suggesting but not proving a causal risk of childhood lymphoma, leukemia and nervous system cancers in those children exposed to magnetic fields from residential 60 Hz electrical power distribution systems. This finding was also supported by adult studies. **These frequencies are thought to be on the low end, however, they are not the 0-30 Hz frequencies that the earth produces found in nature known as the healing frequencies,** and have shown considerable adverse health effects in animal studies. Thus, the 50-60 Hz range have become a major part of the earth's electromagnetic field due to technology and overshadow the earth's natural frequencies on sensitive geomagnetic field tests.

There are the harmful microwave frequencies dominating our technology with a range somewhere between infra-red and radio waves at 2.4 GHz, the primary frequency for: cell phones, cell phone towers, Wi-Fi, Bluetooth, baby monitors, cordless phones and more. Many people are not aware that the bases of cordless phones are constantly emitting harmful frequencies whether or not they are in use. These frequencies are at very powerful intensities - much more powerful than from a cell phone. **(45)**

Microwave technology was developed by the Germans in the 1930s. They used this technology to develop a radar system for early detection of British bombers during WWII. In wintertime, the German soldiers would gather round this radar screen which emitted a great deal of heat to keep them warm. After a short time, many soldiers became very ill and developed leukemia. The Supreme Command of the "Wehrmacht" declared that since human engineered microwaves heat and adversely affect human tissues they should be abandoned. A Berlin University researcher received a grant to develop microwave ovens for war time soldiers to heat their meals. However, like the experience with the radar exposure, many soldiers developed cancer of the blood when they ate the microwaved food. Consequently, microwave ovens were forbidden in the entire Third Reich.

Dr. Hans Herten, a Swiss doctor, was the first scientist to study microwave ovens and found that they have detrimental effects on the human body, such as decreased red and white blood cells as well as hemoglobin production, all of which can be indicative of anemia and poisoning. Under a microscope, blood from healthy persons crystalizes into fine, beautiful crystals. Blood from those eating microwave food crystalizes into a cruciform structure typically seen in patients suffering from cancer. He even concluded that, "There are no atoms, molecules, or cells of any organic system able to withstand such a violent, destructive power for any period of time. This will happen even given the microwave oven's lower power range of milliwatts."

It is common acceptable knowledge now that cell phones have adverse health effects; currently the controversy focuses on the level of danger from exposure. Sleep disturbances have also been shown to occur after an hour of exposure to cell phone use. Women who carry a cell phone in a shirt pocket have shown an increase in breast cancer rates. Another Brazilian study linked 7,000 deaths to cell phone towers.

These EMF's are bad news; they are all around us yet are invisible and have no odor. The public must wake up realize that just like the SAD, with advanced technologies comes health hazards that need to addressed.

These are just a few examples the pernicious factors, part of the toxic soup, if you will, which I have been referring to throughout this book. Again, in the last chapter of this book, I will make recommendations how to reduce your exposure to many of the toxic agents.

When any of these pernicious agents or toxicities disrupt the body's electromagnetic field; it produces a stress response. What this means, for example, if you walk into a very dark movie theater and have trouble seeing an empty seat, after thirty seconds, your pupils will dilate and then you find a seat. Another example is when you are driving and a car pulls out in front of you, your heart starts beating faster. You had no control over your pupils or your heart; these examples were both natural stress responses

FCT treatment entails placing vials of water containing frequencies within the patients invisible bio-energy field to see if vial frequency resonates with the frequency from their problem area, which could be thyroid, peripheral nerves, or any other body part. If this symptomatic area does not match the correct frequency of the vial, the patient will exhibit a stress response;

Wellness in a Toxic World

the patient has no control over this just like the increased pupil dilation and heart rate episodes. Another great example of this stress response is if someone touches a hot stove, his hand pulls away very swiftly. In particular, the stress response I am looking for is a drawing up of the right leg; this is a response of the ANS or autonomic nervous system which controls all of those bodily functions like breathing and digestion that our body automatically continuously performs without our conscious thought. The energy our bodies uses is known as ATP, or adenosine triphosphate. The "vitality" measures the difference between the amount of energy impairment, from the toxin(s), and the amount of cellular resources remaining to perform normal bodily functions. Those burdened with many toxins show a higher degree of stress response and a lower degree of vitality. In other words, if there is no stress response, the legs remain even indicating good vitality.

In my office, when FCT is indicated, the patient fills out an extensive five page questionnaire in advance and drops if off before the appointment. I am looking for different pernicious factors. The form provides a patient's dental history, including the number of amalgam fillings, gold crowns, other metals - how many and how long they have been in the mouth, and whether and when any have been removed. EMF exposure is another important issue to know; how far away are power lines, where do they come into a patient's house, how many computers and televisions are in the house, whether the computer or mouse is wireless, any cordless phones, any bedroom alarm clocks, electric blankets, and any fluorescent lights. The next section of the form contains questions about all the patient's symptoms and they must rate these with key general areas, such as sleep and mood, on a 1-10 scale. After thoroughly studying this questionnaire, I decide which organs are under the most stress and need the most support. I also consider other pernicious factors such as antibiotic residue or radiation as possibly causative.

For the FCT exam I instruct the patient to wear comfortable clothing, preferably cotton and natural fibers without too much bling. I have the patient remove all metal from their body; this includes belts, jewelry etc.. All electronic devices should be turned off prior to entering the treatment room. THE VIALS ARE VERY SENSTIVE TO EMFS; THIS IS VERY IMPORTANT. The patient lies supine (face up) on a very comfortable massage table and I place a conducting rod in their hand with instructions to relax, be still, and to not speak once I begin. Talking will be a distraction to me from the test; if I need to, I will question the patient. Inherently, most patients are so relaxed that they are sound asleep within minutes. The first exam can take up to an hour and follow up exams are usually 30 minutes or so.

When the test is competed, I will go over the results with the patient and make remedies accordingly. These remedies include water vials infused with the frequencies with which the patient's body did not correctly resonate. I also give exact written instructions on how to take these remedies. These consist of 7-12 small dropper bottles. ONE DROP of each remedy in specific order throughout the day for one to two days must be taken. The patient needs to avoid EMFs for two days on average. This means no television, computers, electrical tools, cell/cordless phones, fluorescent lighting, and driving or riding in cars. (A weekend or a couple days in a row off work is the best time to take the remedies). The patient should unplug everything in the bedroom before bedtime. A cell phone can be substituted for an alarm clock if placed on airplane mode not emitting any EMFs. No televisions, computers, or electrical devices should be within 15 feet of the bed; wireless internet should be turned off. I ask the patient to follow as many of these instructions as possible, realizing that they may sound extreme. The reason is that everyone has different levels of EMF sensitivity Thus, these instructions are in place to protect even those patients with the highest sensitivities. Finally, I emphasize the importance of storing the remedy bottles away from any electrical outlets, cell/cordless phones, microwaves, refrigerators, lamps, radios, and computers. Remember, the patient will receive explicit written instructions. There are those patients who will also need to repeat some of the remedies a couple of days to one week later. Most patients are seen on 3-4 week follow ups. Some people will experience quick and dramatic changes. This accompanies feeling very fatigued as the body eliminates toxins and healing begins during this time; this fatigue is only temporary. The majority of patients, however, will make gradual progress. Each treatment will be similar, yet unique from the previous one.

Remember, FCT treatment works on an energetic level, transferring information and affecting the cells with profound changes, which is the driving force to affect cellular chemistry and physiology. Whether or not a patient makes rapid or gradual progress, FCT is a priority based treatment. It will remove toxins from the deepest layers with the body's highest priority in mind. People always want to know how long they should continue their FCT treatment.. The fact that we live in this toxic environment only reinforces my recommendations of at least three to six months of treatment but preferably 12 months. Depending on how a person's symptomatic profile is coupled with their past exposure to toxicity will decide the duration of treatment. Once the initial care plan is successfully completed, patients are advised to come in quarterly or at least yearly, otherwise they runs the risk of repeated toxic buildup, burdened by taking drugs and covering up the symptoms. One of my FCT instructors, Dr. Simon Rees, most accurately described all disease as, "information deficit." He added that "we pace the follow ups to re-checking the systems' (of the body) need for information while whittling away the causes of disease - a process not an event."

The ability of the body's cells to communicate on the energetic level is of profound importance since conventional medical research and thinking on human function, up to this point, has been almost all about hormones, peptides, proteins, and various chemicals that adversely affect bodily functions. Therefore, they prescribe drugs, recommend supplements and/or nutritional recommendations to alter body functions; they only address the body through biochemistry. Therefore **to find answers to the question of cellular health and toxicity, we must speak the language of the body- vibrational/digital medicine/FCT.**

8. Pulsed Electromagnetic Field Therapy (PEMF)

Although many different PEMF (pulsed electromagnetic field therapy) devices have been extensively used for decades in the treatment of many conditions, with over 2,000 peer reviewed studies on "Pub Med," this invaluable therapy remains mostly unknown in the conventional "medical therapy" world. As a matter of fact, I suspect that most of you readers probably have never even heard of PEMF. Recently the National Institutes of Health have made these devices "a priority for research," according to Dr. William Pawluk, a board certified Holistic practitioner, former John Hopkins professor and PEMF expert. He reports that many PEMF devices have already been FDA approved for specific conditions such as to fuse broken bones, for wound healing, for pain and tissue swelling reduction, and to treat depression. PEMF, as the name implies, provides a pulsed magnetic field that is beneficial in supporting the body's natural healing ability. In the article "Zap" by Karl H. Schoenbach, Richard Nuccitelli, and Stephen J. Beebe, they describe the power of certain high intensity PEMF devices: "40 thousand volts, four thousand amperes, and over one hundred million watts squeezed into a cubic centimeter." This surely is enough power to turn most matter into thin air, no? Well, the authors say that, "The trick is to apply that gargantuan jolt for only a few billionths of a second. That's so brief a time that the energy delivered is a mere 1.6 joules per cubic centimeter - barely enough to heat a thimble full of water one third of a degree Celsius." Folks we are talking about only nanoseconds here to turn on and off thousands of volts and amperes of current - the same type of parameters needed to detonate nuclear bombs.

PEMF is based on the fact that humans are electrical beings, the body fluids passing into and out of the cells carry electrical charges. There are optimal charges that need to be maintained for the body to function correctly. <u>Dr. Harold Saxton Burr, professor at Yale University School of Medicine, studied the characteristics of the "bio-magnetic field" associated with living organisms and discovered that imbalances in the cell voltage preceded the onset of disease.</u> He provided solid physical evidence by both electromagnetic measurement and physical appearance demonstration that the body's electromagnetic property was "the organizing principle that kept living tissue from falling into a chaotic state." For example, he showed how disease, cancer in this particular case, occurs after measurable changes in the organism's electrical field. **(46)**

Expanding on the above, we must look at the body's pH. Remember, I previously stressed that the body's body pH should be between 6.4 and 7.4, the body's mineral content, in order for us to maintain good health. I was referring to the mineral content, however, we have to look deeper into what this abbreviation really signifies. **PH stands for potential hydrogens and is really a measure of the body's voltage.** With electrons, there are electron donors and electron stealers, measured with an instrument known as the voltmeter. A positive charge sign in front of a number denotes an electron stealer with that particular number of stealing power. On the other hand a negative sign in front of a number denotes that number of electron donating power. Cellular biology textbooks recommend a normal cell voltage to be between 7.35-7.45 pH. This corresponds logarithmically to a -20 - -25 Mv(millivolts) of electron donor status. (-20 - -25 millivolts is the operating environment and -90 is the gradient for any chemistry gurus out there. So -90 millivolts can be termed normal cell voltage as long as one states whether they are measuring across the cell membrane). Most would agree that an acidic pH is more unfavorable and an alkaline one is good in terms of overall health. The reason is that pH acidity signifies an "electron stealer" status indicating free radicals causing damage. Once a cell steals an electron from another, it damages that cell. The body cells needs to be in a donor, alkaline, status, in order to perform their necessary normal daily functions. This is where the anti-oxidants come in - the dark leafy greens such as kale, collards, and swiss chard; these are loaded with them.

Many patients want to simply measure salivary pH. Keep in mind salivary ph is about .08 pH units less than cellular pH and is not a good indicator because it does not measure the voltage of the fluid around the cells like **urinary** pH does. If we look at cell voltage ranges and how they correspond

Wellness in a Toxic World

to body health and function, we can predict that higher negative cell voltage equates to better health and more work ability. One key to good health is the constant renewal of cells and the cleanup of dead ones. Let's say, for example, I trip on a toy dog and scrape my shin. In order to repair the damage, my body must form a group of new cells. My blood vessels will dilate and raw materials such as the proteins, fats, carbohydrates, and minerals rush in. To turn these raw materials into a scar we need energy. The voltage needed for this task will be -50Mv. When I am healed, the voltage will return to the healthy -20 - -25 Mv range. On the other hand, if the voltage goes below the -20 - -25, the person will feel less than adequate, tired, sick etc. Thus, a person's voltage-pH will constantly be in flux depending on current demand. As one's cell voltage continues to drop, its polarity changes from an electron donor status to that of an electron stealer. When the cell voltage drops and remains there a long time, chronic diseases may result. When it falls down to a +30 millivolts it indicates a very serious chronic disease - possibly even cancer. In this case, the bodies' organs do not have the sufficient energy either to perform normal daily functions or to detoxify all of the toxic soup/waste materials constantly accumulating. To remain and keep healthy, our bodies are in constant need of donor status electrons/voltage. An interesting experiment revealing the importance of voltage to the body, involves placing a tube in a glass of water. When oxygen is bubbled into the water, the amount dissolved is determined by the voltage of the water; the higher the voltage, the more oxygen absorption. Yet, as the voltage drops, the oxygen leaves the water. **(47)** Consider the fact that 75% of the human body is water; this means the cells need to be constantly bathed in oxygen to do their job without incidence. If we examine how the body cells normally get voltage we must look to the Krebs cycle. This is the energy engine in our bodies which performs many chemical reactions and converts fatty acids from the foods we eat into glucose - our source of fuel, like a car using gas. ATP (adenosine triphosphate) is the fuel needed for energy. In the presence of oxygen, our bodies make 38 molecules of ATP for every unit of fatty acids processed through the Krebs Cycle. Yet, if oxygen is not there, only two molecules of ATP are produced from that same amount of fatty acids. How do you think your body will run on this amount of fuel? It is as if your car, now getting 38 miles per gallon of gas, drops to 2. How efficiently is your body going to perform its vital functions? Another problem with a low oxygen situation is that infections/bugs thrive in this acidic, lower pH environment. **Chronic disease looms in the background in this scenario.**

One might ask, "How do our bodies get this much needed voltage?" When discussing the toxic soup, I briefly answered this question. Our style of living in modern society has eliminated most of the natural ways to get voltage. As I said in the FCT chapter, the earth is a large electromagnet; walking barefoot on the grass, for example, infuses our body with necessary electrons and the laws of physics dictate that these electrons flow from areas of higher voltage to areas of lower voltage. Of course walking around shoeless could put us in the Wal-Mart vault of bizarre photography. Today's behavioral standards dictate that we put shoes on when we leave the house. Because so many of us leave the house and go to work in offices or other areas demanding wearing shoes, many of us lack the opportunity to walk directly on the electron rich earth.

Another great source of electrons is ground water. However, a problem arises because most drinking water is loaded with toxic chemicals like chloride and fluoride which turn it from electron donor status to electron stealer status; people drinking tap water are decreasing their own essential voltage. I also must state that raw food measured by a voltmeter will always have more voltage than processed food measured by one. The SAD is contributing to this low voltage status and consequently, inferior health.

Dr. Tennant describes many more interesting examples of electron donors versus stealers. One example, seemingly innocent, is moving air. People are usually more tired after sleeping with a fan blowing on them or riding in a convertible with the top down. "Moving air is an electron stealer." **Some good news: Muscles act as piezoelectric crystals and create electrons when contracting/exercising. Thus movement recharges our batteries. This should motivate us to exercise.**

In addition to the SAD, toxic environmental materials, shoes preventing direct contact with the earth, architectural building materials such as macadam and concrete, and a toxic water supply, all contribute to us getting less voltage than our ancestors.

To describe how our body cells hold and store a charge we must look at how conductors and capacitors work. Dr. Tennent describes this perfectly when he clearly states that "cell membranes serve as battery packs" since "anytime two conductors (opposing phospholipid layers of the cell) are separated by an insulator (legs), you have an electronic device called a capacitor," which is designed to store electrons. These legs of the phospholipids, or unusual fats which make up the cell membranes, can twist like rope to either let light, water, or other molecules into the cell depending on the voltage. From here the discussion gets too complicated; what the reader needs to know is that our body cells hold a charge and that we need to consume plenty of fats (25% at least) to keep making good cells and to store a charge/voltage. The plastic fats or "trans fats" I previously discussed are really one carbon away from plastic and DO NOT HOLD A CHARGE. WITHOUT A CHARGE YOUR CELLS DO NOT HAVE THE NECESSARY ENERGY TO WORK AND THEREFORE THEY CEASE TO LIVE.

I must stress the importance of good, pure water as it is extremely necessary to hold and carry the vital charge needed for life: Unfortunately, pure water is becoming scarce due to all of the chemical toxicity out there. Water in the high surgery and often caffeinated drinks is not acceptable because it does not have the correct charge/pH to contain electrons; this worsened when the toxic elements fluoride and chlorine were added. Pure water is alkaline and an electron donor; toxic loaded water is acidic and an electron stealer. The chemical laden Pepsi and Coke are so highly acidic they will dissolve battery corrosion; unlike pure water, however, they will not hold and carry the proper charge in the body. This clean, pure water is needed not only to carry a charge but to carry away the waste in our bodies. All of these drinks, other than water, do not contain pure water and are not efficient at cleansing the 2000 liters of blood the kidneys must do each day. I tell patients kidney stones may be in their future if they do not drink pure water. Incidentally, if Pepsi and Coke can destroy battery corrosion what must it do to the human digestive system?

Along with water, minerals are needed for all of the body's processes. For example, calcium will cause the contraction of a muscle and another mineral, magnesium, will cause the muscle to relax; many of the muscle cramps people experience are due to a magnesium deficiency. If you think about it, the terms pH and voltage are a measure of the body's mineral content. Please understand, one cannot simply take a variety of minerals and expect to have proper mineral balance.. A majority of people have an acidic pH reflecting this mineral deficiency or imbalance.

There are four ways to charge a body's cell. First we have cellular exercise followed by raw food, natural spring water, and magnetic fields. PEMF therapy is based on the theory that with enough voltage and raw materials, i.e., good water, proper diet, vitamins and minerals, THE BODY CAN HEAL ALMOST ANYTHING.

PEMF exercises the cells and due to its extremely fast short bursts of power has the ability to do what nothing else can, bypass the outside of the cell harmlessly and shock the vital structures of the cell within affecting them mechanically, electrically, chemically and magnetically.

In 1995 two scientists, Siskin and Walker, summarized the clinical results of a study of soft tissue damage treated with PEMF. They reported 10 positive effects with zero adverse side effects. The conclusion was a significant decrease in pain. Many studies over the years, some short term, some longer, recorded the same significant decrease in pain. One study, performed at the Madigan Army Medical Center, Tacoma, Washington in particular, was a double blind placebo controlled study on PEMF and the treatment of migraine headaches. This study evaluated 42 subjects who met the International Headache Society's criteria. Of the 73% receiving actual PEMF treatment, 45% saw a substantial decrease and 14% an excellent decrease in headaches. They gave half of those receiving actual PEMF exposure 2 more weeks of treatment. All of them showed a 50% substantial decrease and a 38% excellent decrease. They concluded that exposure to PEMF for at least 3 weeks is an effective short term intervention for migraines. **(48)**

With PEMF's effects on traumatically injured tissue, a study done by Jorgensen W. at the International Pain Research Institute in California, concluded that, "Unusually effective and long - lasting relief of pelvic pain of gynecological origin has been obtained consistently by short exposures of affected areas to the application of a magnetic induction device. Treatments are short, fast-acting, economical, and in many instances have obviated surgery." The study showed that patients suffering from endometriosis, pre-menstrual syndrome, ruptured ovarian cyst, acute urinary infection, dyspareunia (painful intercourse) who did not receive pain medication were treated with PEMF and "90% of the patients experienced marked, even dramatic relief, while 10% reported less than complete pain. **(49)**

A study was done by Kaan Uzunca, Murat Birtane, and Nuretin Tastekin at Trakya University Medical Faculty and Physical Medicine and Rehabilitation Department in Edirne, Turkey on the effectiveness of PEMF against sham PEMF and steroid injection for lateral epicondylitis, also known as tennis elbow. Patients with epicondylitis were randomly, equally distributed into three groups. One group received actual PEMF, another sham PEMF, and the last a cortisone injection. Pain at rest, activity, during nighttime, with resisted bending of the wrist up and down, and with forearm resistance in wrist down and wrist up positions, were determined with a visual analog scale form. And an algometer, which measures how much force is applied by the examiner, measured the pain threshold. All patients were evaluated three weeks before treatment and three months later. "Pain levels were significantly lower in the group treated with the local steroid at the third week, but the group treated with PEMF had lower pain during rest, activity and nighttime than the group receiving steroids at the third month." **(50)**

PEMF has shown to be effective for both short and long term pain reduction, reducing inflammation, increasing cellular flexibility and increasing circulation. I will simplify this to make it more easily understandable. The voltage difference between the exterior and interior of the cell is known as the trans-membrane potential or TMP. Ions, or charged minerals in different concentrations on opposite sides of the cellular membrane produce this TMP. The most prevalent ions are Na+ and Cl- ions on the outside of the cell or extracellular and K+ ions on the inside or intracellular region. When the channels of these ions are opened or closed the TMP changes resulting in rapid electric current flow to various points of the cellular membrane. With a change in the TMP, a chemical transmitter is released and transferred across the synaptic gap, the gap between pre and post or before and after nerve reaction. This all happens in $1/2000^{th}$ of a second. So in other words, a pain signal arrives and the TMP of the cell goes from -70 millivolts to +30 millivolts a process known as depolarization. During this time, the ion channels are opening and ions are shifting around. Once the process is complete, the cell must depolarize to its resting -70 millivolts. Research by Warnke et al , 1983 and 1997, established that the application of PEMF therapy has an effect that "hyperpolarizes" the -70 millivolts to -90 millivolts and when the repolarization with the pain signal occurs the TMP only raises to +10 millivolts, well below the needed +30 millivolts necessary to release the pain blocking chemicals, and the pain signal is effectively blocked. **Thus by causing a hyperpolarized state at the TMP, PEMF therapy effectively blocks pain by preventing the threshold necessary to transmit the pain signal to be reached.**

Reducing inflammation reduces pain. A New York University Medical Center study at the Institute of Reconstructive Plastic Surgery NY, NY, "demonstrates that electro-magnetic fields increased angiogenesis." The researchers found that with fractures, direct application of PEMF did not heal it with osteogenesis (formation of new bone cells); instead, it was a result of the increased vascularity (angiogenesis), and the fact that PEMF augments the interaction between osteogenesis and blood vessel growth.

It has been established that PEMF affects the trans-membrane potential (TMP) and the flow of ions in and out of the cell, as I previously stated, by accelerating the re-establishment of the normal TPM voltage. This process accelerates healing and decreases swelling. Dr. Thomas Valone, demonstrated that diseased or damaged cells have an unusually low TPM voltage - 80% lower than healthy cells; this adversely affects the normal sodium/potassium pump necessary for the body's ATP energy production. Normally there is a ratio of 3 sodium ions pumped out of the cell for every 2 potassium ions pumped into it needed for proper metabolism. If this ratio does not occur, a poor functioning sodium/potassium pump will result in cellular water accumulation, known as edema or swelling. This could then lead to a process called fermentation, which is favorable towards cancerous activity. Dr. Albert Szent-Gyorgyi established, in 1976, that PEMF stimulates the TMP which is, "proportional to the activity of the sodium/potassium pump and thus to the rate of healing."

In a study "Modulation of collagen production in cultured fibroblasts by a low-frequency magnetic field." Murray et.al, **(51)** found that when PEMF cultured cells were treated for 24 hours and 6 days, these cells exhibited a collagen production increase compared to total protein indicating that PEMF "can specifically increase collagen production." Thus, PEMF also increases cellular flexibility due to this collagen synthesis leading to
tissue and muscle flexibility, and therefore, a rapid increase in range of motion.

In 1984, a study on DNA synthesis by low intensity magnetic fields, Liboff and Rosch et.al., discovered that proteins are conductors of electricity and when exposed to strong fields, these protein molecules will start to separate. The RNA messengers that are made from the DNA template will mediate the transfer of genetic information from the center of the cell or the nucleus of the cell to other parts of the cell and serve as a template for protein synthesis. Thus, PEMF stimulates cellular communication and replication.

PEMF therapy also restores order in a disordered organ or tissue. Since each organ and tissue have its own frequency, if one does not resonate at the proper frequency, a disruption in the magnetic resonance of the electrons occurs - a phase shift, which "disturbs and breaks the once orderly pathways of communication that is usually transmitted from atom to molecule, molecule to cell and tissue to organ."

In dealing with PEMF treatment and the spine, there is a important long term study, "Spine fusion for discogenic low back pain: outcome in patients treated with or without pulsed electromagnetic field stimulation." **(52)** This study included 61 laminectomy fusion patients who had failed to respond to preoperative conservative treatment for their discogenic pain. The fusion succeeded in 97.6% of the 42 patients who underwent PEMF stimulation, and only 52.6% of the 19 patients who did not receive electrical stimulation of any kind.

Moreover, PEMF has shown great results in the management of rotator cuff tendonitis. The department of rheumatology at Addenbrookes Hospital, Cambridge England, conducted a trial in the use of PEMF therapy for the treatment of "persistent rotator cuff tendonitis." They applied PEMF to those showing no relief from steroid injection and other conventional treatments. "At the end of the trial, 65% of these were symptom free, with 18% of the remainder being greatly improved."

Another area showing promise with PEMF treatment is food sensitivities. (A true "allergy" is an immune cell response which occurs for a multitude of reasons and involves biochemical reactions. The PEMF treatment does not erase allergies). On the other hand, "sensitivities" involve energetic stresses. A person may be under a lot of emotional, chemical or physical stress that becomes unbearable and leads to an exaggerated response. This results in a symptom(s) such as a runny nose, watery eyes, cough, dizziness, digestive or intestinal discord etc.. Many logical thinkers will simply say, "Avoid the offending food or substance and it will not bother you." The problem with this thinking, however, is that smelling or touching the offending substance, can evoke a serious sharp reaction. This can really adversely affect one's social life and livelihood. PEMF utilizes a method for removing many patients food sensitivities. You must REMEMBER, however, this does not now make the former offending food or substance good for you; it only makes you not react to it. Some doctors in my forum group have also had success using this protocol to rid patients of pet sensitivities.

A recent, fascinating German study on the brain and PEMF treatment, a 4 week double-blind, placebo-controlled study was conducted in Munich, Germany by Uni der Bundeswehr evaluating the efficiency of PEMF treatment for insomnia. One hundred and one subjects were given either active PEMF treatment or placebo and were placed into one of three diagnostic groups: sleep latency, interrupted sleep, or nightmares. Of those actually receiving PEMF treatment, 70% or 34 of the patients experienced substantial or even complete relief of their complaints; 24% or 12 patients reported clear improvement; 6% or 3 patients noted a slight improvement. Of the placebo patients, only 2% had very clear relief; 49% or 23 patients saw no change in their symptoms. **No adverse effects of the treatment were reported.** Another study, "Protection against focal cerebral ischemia following exposure to a pulsed electro-magnetic field," by Dr G. Grant of the Department of Neurosurgery at Stanford University, showed some incredible encouraging results for stroke victims. He found that PEMF stimulation may accelerate the healing of tissue damage following lack of blood flow to the cortical areas of the brain, which receive and process information and control behavior. He stated that this was evidenced on MRI showing a 65% reduction in brain edema or swelling.

Finally, there is a study conducted by Sandyk R. on the topic of Multiple Sclerosis, a devastating disease that is the third most common cause of severe disability in patients between 15 and 50 years of age. This is a disease of the central nervous system (brain and spinal cord) whose cause is unknown; the disease causes a demyelination of the covering of nerves so they cannot smoothly communicate with each other. This results in some of the following symptoms: central fatigue, impaired bladder control, muscle weakness, sensory deficits, impaired cognition (learning disability), among others. Sandyk R. published a summary of his recent work on the therapeutic effects of PEMF on Multiple Sclerosis. He noted that there has been no treatment, other than PEMF which will restore the neurons to their pre - MS diseased state. Interactions between genetics, the immune system, the environment, and hormonal factors cannot be explained by demyelination alone, according to Sandyk. He added that there must be some crucial area that has not been investigated and concluded that this pivotal area is the pineal gland; this gland functions as a magneto-receptor organ which is therefore very receptive to "PEMF's flux density (strength of an electric field as electrons pass through it) as a highly effective therapeutic modality."

To summarize, PEMF really stimulates/exercises the body cells which then promotes cellular metabolism which in turn promotes tissue regeneration and immune system response; then finally, you guessed it, maintains general health. In my clinic, I have seen some miraculous results using PEMF. For example, a woman who could barely walk, due to severe lower back pain incurred the previous night, came to my clinic. I decided to try PEMF because she could not even lie on a table. I have a chair with my PEMF machine and sat her down for 50 minutes at a frequency of 1 hertz - the indicated frequency for an acute painful condition. My patient hardly felt the intensity of the treatment. The next day she called and told Becky that she was 98% better. I have been currently treating a middle aged patient who had lower back fusion surgery, with rods and pins inserted, that eventually broke and were removed years ago. He has been complaining of severe lower back pain for many years and after 6 visits, he said this is the first time in thirty years that he could stand up straight.. He stated, "I have not felt this good since I was in my thirties." I have had elderly patients who love the energy boost they get with PEMF. There have been chronic headache patients who had their headaches reduced by 80%. I had a 70 year old woman who had a constant migraine headache for a month. We gave her a free treatment and she called Becky the next day only to say it was the first time in a month she did not wake up with the headache. She said she had "tried everything." One gentleman I treated had a knee replacement that was not a total success. The PEMF restored his flexibility when three months of physical therapy failed to do so. Personally, I have had success with eliminating the need to get up in the middle of the night to go to the bathroom. After discussing this with many of my colleagues on the Johnson board, we all agree, PEMF seems to decrease inflammation of the prostate and takes pressure off the bladder. To maintain my positive results, I do one 30 minute PEMF maintenance visit every week. **All men over 40 should do a series of at least 10 hours of treatment followed by weekly maintenance sessions to keep their prostate healthy. If you do nothing, the current odds for getting prostate cancer are one out of two!**

Viewing the Johnson board this past week, I noticed that a colleague actually bought a microscope and took a drop or two of patients' blood before and after PEMF treatment to compare it. After the comparison of the two slides, before and after treatment, it is immediately visible that the red blood cells pre-PEMF treatment were abnormally clumped together. This can result, for example, from sitting in front of a computer or having a cell phone right against the body, both causes of the "electrosmog" I previously mentioned. As a result of this dirty electricity, the cells clump together and lose their ability to hold a charge or bind to oxygen effectively. Consequently, these clumped cells then had trouble passing into the capillaries to dump off oxygen and nutrients - a very unhealthy state. Immediately after treatment, viewing another slide of their blood, the cells were now normally noticeably spaced apart indicating their ability to now hold a charge and bind to oxygen; this is the favorable healthy state.

In my office, a typical PEMF treatment entails a specific package of visits. Remember, aside from any symptoms many people use the PEMF as a wellness treatment to maintain a healthy cellular charge. Before treatment, a patient signs a release form which states the only contraindications excluding him from PEMF treatment. It includes the following: **DO NOT USE PEMF IF YOU ARE PREGNANT OR HAVE: ANY IMPLANTED MEDICAL DEVICES SUCH AS PACEMAKERS, DEFIBRILLATORS, COHCLEAR DEVICES AND INSULIN PUMPS.** Prior to a treatment, people must empty their pockets and remove any car keys, hearing aids, cell phones and jewelry.

The visit consists of a total of 50 minutes. First off, we have the patient do a four minute warm-up along the governor meridian, the main energetic pathway, which runs down the center of the body. Next, depending the nature of the problem I may split the treatment into two sessions of 23 minutes, or three sessions of 15 minutes and move the applicators around. Often, the patient will just remain in the same position with the applicator(s) in the same configuration during the entire duration of the treatment. At this time, the patient will also feel a sensation of tingling, throbbing, or mild pain depending on the chosen strength of the magnetic field used. The location where the patient feels the magnetic pulse the strongest correlates with their lowest areas of cellular energy. Sometimes Becky or I will do a pre-treatment scan to discover areas of low energy the patient is unaware of because they have no overt symptoms there.

Most people decide to continue after the first free visit and have questions about the treatment schedule. Research has shown that the ideal amount of time, in hours, needed to build the body's electrical foundation so that it can begin to repair and regenerate is at least 10 hours but preferably 30 to 48 hours. Remember, when the body is ill, injured or has a chronic disease, the cells need 2-5 times as much energy to heal. Many patients ask how long the body will hold a charge; that is a good question because cells need good nutrients, minerals, and water (like the chemicals in a battery) to hold a charge. THEREFORE, THE BETTER YOUR NUTRITION, INCLUDING PINK SEA SALT AND GOOD MINERAL WATER CONSUMPTION, THE LONGER YOUR BODY WILL HOLD A CHARGE. Before each treatment, the body MUST be hydrated so I give a patient an 8 ounce cup of water mixed with minerals to ensure good conduction and charge hold. How long the body holds a charge, along with pain relief duration is also proportional to the health of the cell. Less healthy individuals will need more treatment over time.

FOR All PATIENTS STARTING TREATMENT THE SCHEDULE IS THREE VISITS PER WEEK UNTIL 10 HOURS ARE REACHED, USUALLY 12 VISITS; THEN THEY CAN BE RE-ASSESED. We offer 12 visit, 30 visit, and 48 visit packages, as well as a maintenance package of 2-4 hours per month.

Some patients ask whether a person can do too much PEMF therapy? The answer is yes during a treatment; sometimes the treatment duration and intensity for certain weaker-nutritionally compromised patients might exceed the persons metabolic capacity to process it, resulting in their getting sore or light headed. Consider a person with poor diet, water intake, etc. whose circulation may also not be optimal. Imagine how this patient will feel when PEMF gives a huge boost to the body's circulation with all of the blood vessels dilating? I find that another session the next day at a very low setting will set things straight again; it simply means that the patient's compromised body could not tolerate the initial level of treatment. As far as receiving too much PEMF treatment in terms of too many visits, the answer is never. It is simply energy, your body will soak it up like a sponge.

Think of it this way. Part of living in toxic soup consists of AC (alternating current), man made dirty electricity and harmful electro-magnetic frequencies, such as cell phones, their towers, wireless internet, and computers, which interfere with our normal biofeild. As stated in previous chapters, just by living in a modern technologically advanced society, we are constantly being exposed.

This modality, like the k-laser I discussed in my last book, is a stand - alone treatment. However, unlike the laser, PEMF treatment does not have to applied against the bare skin making its application much broader.

I cannot stress the serious healthful effects of this fantastic cutting edge technology. In closing this chapter, I want to compare the human body to a battery. When afflicted with a chronic health condition, the body is like a corroded battery holding little charge which diminishes as time passes. PEMF will re-charge that battery allowing that body to perform at it's optimum level. Because, I am so confident about the effectiveness of this therapy, **I OFFER EVERYONE A FREE INITIAL VISIT.**

9. Nature's Gem Gone Awry: The Immune System

There is so much to say about the immune system. Let me begin by saying that it is the most misunderstood and underestimated body system, yet it plays a vital major role in all of the increasingly prevalent chronic diseases currently ravaging our country. Most people erroneously believe they have a certain disease, but in reality they have an autoimmune disease that results from the contemporary lifestyle including, childhood vaccinations, flu vaccines, pesticides, dirty electricity exposure, and the SAD among others; the toxic soup. All of these factors adversely affect the gut barriers, which houses most of the immune system, by causing gaps or holes in which, parasites and undigested food particles, for example, can get through; these then will elicit an immune response. This process is known as "leaky gut syndrome." When these barriers are strong, they only allow immune cells through to perform normal necessary maintenance functions such as clearing dead cells. However, when these barriers grow weak or porous, due to the aforementioned factors, they lead to adrenal malfunction, poorly regulated blood sugar levels, gut infections, and chronic stress. This results in an overworked immune system on overtime. It must try and stop intruders from getting in through the leaky pores from every direction, **but** it starts to attack everything including the body tissue, creating massive chronic inflammation and serious symptoms.

The immune system is designed to kill unwanted intruders like bacteria or viruses for example, living organisms that are foreign and harmful to the body known as bio-toxins.

At this point, I must explain only the major players in this complex, crucial immune system. In addition to the barriers in the gut, there are also some in the respiratory tract and the brain (i.e. the blood brain barrier) which can all become leaky. An entire immune response is initially set off by an ANTIGEN; this is a foreign invader that could be a toxic heavy metal like mercury, for example. First, a macrophage cell or a large white blood cell eats and envelops the invading antigen known as an APC (antigen presenting cell). These cells are the first responders, like the paramedics to the accident scene, and they sound the alarm for the remaining players in the immune system. Next we have the T-helper cells who then send messengers known as cytokines to the cellular hit men known as the TH1 system: Natural killer cells and Cytotoxic T cells swarm the enemy antigen and destroy them. These cytokine messenger cells are also sent to cells known as B-Lymphocytes which identify the antigen and then make antibodies to that antigen like a biologist tags an animal. These B-Lymphocytes store all of the information about the antigen so that if they ever encounter it again, the Natural killer cells and Cytotoxic T cells can kill it. Finally, there are also T-regulator cells and T-suppressor cells that monitor the attack. When the threat is neutralized, these cells tell the whole system that the threat is gone and calms down the immune system returning it to its normal state. Thus these elite killer cells depend on the B-Lymphocyte cells to identify the enemy.

Let's further discuss heavy metal toxicity in Hashimoto's disease, the most common autoimmune disorder involving the thyroid. Mercury is all around us in this toxic world; mainly from vaccinations, fish, amalgam fillings, and fluorescent lights; we are constantly exposed on a regular basis. Toxins which are unable to be cleared or de-toxified by the liver, are delegated to storage in fat cells so the body can be protected from them. Remember, the immune system is only designed to kill living ORGANISMS NOT NON LIVING TOXIC CHEMICALS. **(53)** Thus, it has no chance against the metal; it is not alive. But the body's Th1 cells will keep trying anyway often even forming antibodies (Th2) against the surrounding healthy tissue; in the case of Hashimotos, this will be thyroid tissue. (As a side note, autoimmune conditions are named for the tissues they attack. For example, besides Hashimotos attacking the thyroid tissue, diabetes attacks the pancreas, multiple sclerosis attacks the myelin sheath or covering of the nerves). Thus, a lot of collateral damage will result from this autoimmune attack. This is really just a case of mistaken identity. The body thinks it is doing the right thing and will keep trying to kill like the terminator unless it thinks it finally did. Thus, YOU MUST ATTEMPT TO REMOVE THE ANTIGEN CAUSING THE BODY TO ATTACK ITSELF. It is not enough to keep supporting the tissue under attack quelling any symptoms.

This is like attempting to fill a cracked bucket with water by continually emptying it when the water reaches the damaged level; the bucket needs a patch, right? This is common sense stuff here folks. Returning to the Hashimotos dilemma, simply supporting the thyroid with hormone replacing drugs such as Synthroid does nothing to stop the antigen attack; THE ANTIGEN IS THE CAUSE NOT BEING ADDRESSED. Dr. Kevin Conners in his book, *Stop Fighting Cancer* explains what is actually going on with the thyroid when the patient's doctor wants to increase the meds dosage, for example, on a patient's next visit. While this patient erroneously reasons they have become attenuated to the dosage and just needs more, the actual reason for the increase is that the attacking antigen has destroyed more thyroid tissue since their last visit. Remember, diet is crucial in thyroid conditions. If a thyroid patient eats gluten, for example, the immune system not only attacks the thyroid tissue whose molecular structure is almost identical to the thyroid gland, but also attacks the thyroid because heavy metals are stored there. When the thyroid is attacked, the patient will have more energy because their TSH, is closer to, if not in, the normal range. They will be normal or in a hyperthyroid state with more energy; only temporary, however. Because when metabolized, the TSH will fall far below the normal levels and the patient will be in a hypothyroid-sluggish state. These are the highs and lows of Hashimoto's. I RECOMMNED FINDING A HOLISTIC MEDICAL DOCTOR WHO CAN PROVIDE NATURAL THYROID ALTERNATIVES. It is all about balance between the Th1 and Th2 components of the immune system; picture them on a seesaw continuously going up and down. Suppose a Hashimotos patient goes on a sugar binge for the holidays. This results in extremely high blood sugar leading to leaky gut syndrome allowing an antigen such as bacteria, for example, into the bloodstream. Now the body must try to kill this antigen using the macrophages, the Th1, and Th2 system. Research has shown that MOST AUTO-IMMUNE DISORDERS ARE TH1 DOMINANT: THEIR NATURAL KILLER AND CYCTOXIC T CELLS ARE GOING CRAZY WHILE THEIR T2 B-LYMPHOCYTE CELLS ARE SUPPRESSED. Thus, the immune system must be balanced or modulated to keep the auto-immune disorder in remission. During an auto-immune response to a heavy metal antigen, for example, TH1 will keep trying to kill it. Some people lack T-suppressor cells that tell them to stop the attack. Collateral damage has a greater chance of occurring the longer the attack continues. There are two messengers, IL2 and IL4, which deploy the natural killer cells, cytotoxic T cells, and B-Lymphocyte cells. Some people have too much of these messengers causing too many attacks and therefore too much collateral damage to innocent tissue. In addition, parasites and viruses could also cause IL2 and IL4 to be overproduced. Surprisingly, however, a high carbohydrate diet, the SAD, causes insulin surges which will also stimulate overproduction of B-Lymphocyte cells. Remember, the Th1 pathway is an immediate response, and the Th2 pathway is the delayed response, but both keep attacking and cause the teeter-totter to tip to one side and produce chronic symptoms. **(54)** Dr. Kevin Connors explains this so well in his cancer book that I will quote him, "Usually people with an autoimmune disease that involves a lot of destruction and therefore a lot of symptoms has a Th1 dominant disorder, that is, the immune response is stuck in a Th1 attack. This typically brings about much tissue damage, much inflammation and a greater number of symptoms that causes them to seek medical care and arrive at a diagnosis. They eventually know they have MS, RA, Hashimotos, etc. But the same process that may leave an individual 'stuck' in a Th2 dominant situation often produces a slower attack on tissue, lesser symptoms, a suppressed Th1 response and a chronic, undiagnosed condition. This can lead to secondary conditions from a suppressed Th1 response - cancer."

Besides the Th1 and Th2 there are also Th17 lymphocytes which activate Nitric Oxide Synthase, an enzyme which causes cells to go through apoptosis or programmed cell death. This is due to the lack or failure of the Regulatory T cell system in charge of the entire immune response.

To regulate this imbalance, obviously a patient must avoid as much of the "toxic soup" as possible and try to adopt therapies to balance the immune system so the teeter totter remains level. With most autoimmune disorders, it is necessary to first decrease the antigenic load by reducing food triggers. We can send a patient's blood to Cyrex labs and be very specific on what foods they should avoid, or patients can adopt my autoimmune eating plan for three months which includes avoiding all of the triggers. We can also send patients for a leaky gut test. The second step is to balance the Th1 and Th2 systems and determine which is dominant; then choose nutrition to support it. This could be confusing sometimes depending on the nature of the patient's autoimmune disorder. For example, with cancer, one might reason that nature's best antioxidant, glutathione, would really destroy all of the uncontrolled free radical activity. Ironically, however, if taken by cancer sufferers, it interferes with other substances they may be taking, such as curcumin, whose action is inhibiting cancer growth. Thus, a patient really needs to understand how supplements interact with each other; they may have the opposite dangerous effect. The third step to regulate immunity is to increase the stability of the Regulatory T cells. This includes evaluating Vitamin D levels from bloodwork. Furthermore, other important tests include methylation pathways from the genetic testing and evaluation of the key essential fatty acids are also the key. Finally, the fourth step in the treatment plan is to modulate the T17 activity to decrease activation of cell destruction.

10. What To Do: Applying All Of This To Life

Here we are at the final chapter. Although I had initially intended to amend my first book, after some consideration, I decided that the new services and therapies our office provides, along with the new advances in scientific research, warranted a separate book. While I have repeated some vital material more than once, I am hoping that since repetition is a learning device, you will retain some useful, factual information necessary for a healthy lifestyle. I implore my readers to investigate his or her own health concerns. Obviously, with today's vast social media networks, this can be daunting and overwhelming. Almost daily we read about new drugs on the market, some of which are soon subject to lawsuits and removed from sales, new short drug trials, contradictory information to diet, new exercise guidelines, and increasing use of modified food advertisement. Keep in mind drug advertisers pay millions of dollars to television stations to push their products, and the unsuspecting viewer could easily fall prey to ad's cinematic quality. Remember, money makes the world go around but it also tarnishes the conscience of many. Moreover, large lobbies, like the farmers' for example, pay millions to promote their products, most of which support the SAD; wheat, soybean, corn, and milk.

My original advice from book one still stands on how to apply the information I discussed in detail to regain and maintain health; furthermore, it now contains evidence of new research and additional therapies to supplement it.

As an exercise junky, who has been working out five days per week since I was 15 years old - 35 years ago, I firmly believe that we must keep moving until we die. Resistance training is the best since it builds lean muscle which will stoke the furnace (speed up our metabolism) and help maintain a healthy weight, but should be accompanied some cardio at least three times per week or so for 20-30 minutes to get the heart rate up; even walking is great exercise. The key to exercise and good health is consistency. Unfortunately, however, the **only thing that most people are consistent with, is a lack of consistency**. Most people will not do anything or take any action step towards getting healthier unless they are motivated by a health scare or a social incentive, like a high school re-union, wedding, etc. Very few Americans are willing to sacrifice much to get better; as one of my friends said, "we want what we want when we want it." I understand that most people are raised with varying ideas of what healthy eating entails. Remember, in chapter 3, all of the hidden sugars in the average American's daily diet? My point is that most foods making up **this** SAD are highly processed, full of sugar and hydrogenated fats - that are only one carbon away from plastic!!

For those who want to clean up their diets, my recommendation is to replace non - nutritious foods, one at a time, with better choices. Just change a little at a time so that you do not feel as if you are sacrificing too much; after a while it becomes second nature. For example, in the morning you can at least replace your cold cereal, donuts or Danish with steel cut unsweetened oatmeal. (I recommend making sure it is gluten free - not cross contaminated). To avoid the high carbohydrate food however, it would be better to eat eggs any style with organic bacon containing no nitrates. If you must have potatoes with your eggs, purple or sweet potatoes have a much lower glycemic index (turn to sugar slower) than white potatoes. Eating the oatmeal or too many carbohydrates such as potatoes with the eggs, causes some spikes in blood sugar and you will not be satiated as long as if you ate protein and fat containing foods. Fat and protein meals and snacks will maintain a balanced blood sugar and more even appetite. For snacks I recommend nuts or flourless baked bars. **Sometimes these are referred to as "bread" but the flour is usually almond, tapioca, or coconut - not bread at all.** You can also eat some meat for breakfast with a few strawberries or stone and pitted fruits, which are lower in sugar. Other choices are a green shake in the morning consisting of some kale, swiss chard, spinach, collards or some other dark green leafy vegetable full of vitamins and minerals. (I will put many recipes at the end of this chapter and a sample green shake recipe will be included). The choices depend on whether you are trying to eat healthier or if you are trying to lose weight. If the latter, you must keep your simple carbohydrate ingestion to a minimum. When you do not limit carbohydrates your body will burn them for fuel instead of your own body fat. This is the basis of the ketogenic diet plan I offer known as the T360 plan. If just trying to eat healthier, however, you can have some more carbohydrates but still must eat more complex ones such as the green leafy vegetables, sweet or purple potatoes and long grain brown rice.

As previously stated, **SATURATED FAT IS ACTUALLY GOOD FOR US;** trans-fats or hydrogenated fats are the culprits. Do not worry about having to give up red meat unless you are diagnosed with cancer due to the meat's glutamine content. (This is an amino acid which cancer cells love and use as a transport of nitrogen for protein synthesis of new cancer cells. Wheat is another great source of glutamine as is dairy, except for cottage cheese). Animal products are the best sources of Vit A and D. If you are not in the sun and use sunscreen when you are, and you are a vegetarian, your Vit A and D levels can be too low. Non animal sources of Vit A is olive oil and for Vit D is mushrooms. The precursor to Vit A is beta carotene which must be obtained from fruits and vegetables but still must be converted. Those who happen to have a sluggish thyroid, diabetes, or Celiac's disease will have a much harder time converting it. Now keep in mind that opinions vary on the vegetarian dilemma. "The China Study" published in 2005 consisting of hundreds of thousands of subjects came to the conclusion that those who were vegetarians lived much longer. T Colon Campbell, emeritus professor at Cornell University and the study's main author, boldly stated that, "eating any food with cholesterol levels above 0 mg is unhealthy." There is a lot of controversy concerning this study and his vilification of casein, a milk protein used in the study. One cannot deny the incredible health benefits of plants; they resonate with the same frequencies as the human body as animal products do not. All of PRL products are from plant sources. However, if we look at the cave man diet, today known as the Paleo diet, from the beginning, meat was a staple of the diet. If meat and animal products were bad for human health, wouldn't man have been a vegetarian from the beginning? In today's society that includes all of the toxic soup, especially the SAD containing an incredibly high consumption of animal products and virtually no vegetables, adversely affecting human health, it is not that simple to just say, "Avoid all animal products, eat only vegetables, and go about business as usual." Furthermore, perhaps the greatest justification in the disagreement with "The China Study's" conclusion lies in the fact that it does not address individuality; it does not take into account each person's unique biochemistry and genetics. When some people attempted to "go vegetarian" and exclude all meat, they became lethargic and got sick often. Conversely, when adding animal protein back in their diet, their energy levels skyrocketed and they became sick less often. Also, "The China Study" did not include all organic greens, you have to figure in all of the pesticides which then open the environmental toxicity discussion. The meat is not the problem in the SAD if organic, it is the other components. Thus, the vegetarian diet may be acceptable for many people who feel the best on it as long as they consume the proper nutrients and avoid as much of the toxic soup as they can.

To those with diagnosed cancer it is also suggested not to consume any red meat, organic or not due to it being an acidic food. In their case being more vegetarian is advised. I agree with a large consumption of green leafy vegetables for their mineral content, pH raising ability, and heavy metal detoxification abilities. However, if you can manage your pH and eat red meat and other acidic foods moderation then I think that is the way to live your life. **Due to the prevalence of GMO AND PESTICIDES WITH NON-ORGANIC FOODS, I ONLY RECOMMEND ALL ORGANIC FOODS.**

Thus, in my opinion, the Mediterranean diet is the best but then again I love seafood and nuts. I previously discussed supplement recommendations in book one; therefore, I will only discuss new information about them here.

As an example I will discuss the following supplements that I take daily. Because my gene test showed a heterozygous SNP, every few months I cycle in PRL's Xenostat, a natural form of iodine for the thyroid. It is a natural form Iodine. I inherited the gene trait from one parent prone to thyroid issues. Next I take a teaspoon of Canadian golden honey with Premier Wildland pollen for liver health to keep it clear of toxic build-up. I also mix some ionic minerals and mineral salts from Immunologic in a water bottle to sip throughout the day to maintain a normal pH or mineral content of at least 6.4-7.4. My regimen also includes PRL's Digest, HCL, and HCL Activator two to three times per day or whenever meat, eggs, or dairy (animal protein) is part of the meal. This is because I am fifty and produce less digestive enzymes and less stomach acid than I used to. These three comprise the HCL detox kit. The HCL activator to re-methylate the cells. Six drops of PRLs Vit D with limonene oil emulsifies the Vit D, essential for maintaining immunity, and is responsible for allowing normal cell death - something we do not see in cancer. (Because cholesterol is the raw materials for hormones, and Vit D is a hormone, and with one out of every three adult Americans on a statin/cholesterol lowering drugs, we have a huge problem). With the Vit D, I mix in a quarter of a teaspoon of Max Stress B, and Green Tea ND, both PRL products. The Max Stress B keeps the bile salts in suspension to maintain healthy liver function. For a woman with a history of birth control pills, Max Stress B is essential as the pill permanently necessitates a need to take Vitamin B. PRL's form is the best I have ever found. Green Tea ND supports the parathyroid against heavy metal toxicity. I also rub a drop of dōTERRA's granddaddy of oils,

Frankincense, directly on my head for immune support. Finally, I take dōTERRA's Cellular Vitality and Food Nutrient Complexes in the morning and at night to get those nutrients from a combination of herbs and oils you cannot get from foods alone!

In the morning, after a workout, I drink a green protein shake, containing greens, apple cider vinegar, flax or chia seeds, bananas, coconut oil and some form of protein. Greens are mother nature's best chelators of heavy metals; mercury is the most prevalent. On the five days per week I work out, I eat buckwheat after the shake, a gluten free grain, and I mix in it fruit, coconut milk, wildland pollen and Canadian golden honey. On weekends when I do not work out, I eat a three or four egg omelet with purple potatoes and broccoli. I do not strictly follow the total Paleo because my intension is not to lose weight, however, I mainly keep the starches to complex carbs.

Lunch usually consists of a mixture of ground turkey and chicken with a lot of spices and a sweet potato, and either broccoli, green beans, or Brussel sprouts, plus an apple. Some examples for supper are: gluten free panko chicken, lemon chicken with capers, spaghetti squash, beef with cabbage and salmon. My side dish usually consist of long grain brown rice or purple potatoes. For a vegetable, I also eat broccoli, green beans, cauliflower, squash, broccoli soup, or brussel sprouts. I also try to eat a salad with every supper, which consists of mixed greens, cucumbers, onions, roasted peppers, olives, tomatoes, and a little feta goat cheese; and no iceberg lettuce tossed with Bragg's Vinaigrette or Ginger Sesame dressing. Most salad dressings are nutritionally poor loaded with sugars, soy, preservatives, and contain too many unwanted ingredients, so read the labels carefully. I also drink a cup of bone broth every day, either chicken or beef. I will discuss bone broth shortly, both how to make it and it's benefits. **I must digress from my diet here and add to my previous discussion on fatty acids**. Every day, I also take a key fatty acid omega 3 plant source DHA from PRL, which is tremendously benefit to the brain, nervous system, eyes, heart and lungs. Importantly, this is sourced form algae instead of fish. I agree with this vegetarian source because the quality of most fish oils sold is poor and quickly turns rancid. In processing the fish oil, many companies use molecular distillation which alters the molecular weights of the original oils in such a way that the natural beneficial triglycerides are lost. These altered oils require more distillation to separate into alcohols and then fatty acids. Farm raised salmon, for example, is not an acceptable source because it is fed un-natural food and is GMO. Considering the fact that the fish is the middleman who feed on the algae, why not just cut out the middleman (fish) and go right to the source? Among the numerous studies showing the many health benefits of omega-3 fatty acids, one recent Finnish study showed that the serum blood level of CRP (c-reactive protein), a marker for inflammation, was inversely proportional to omega-3 fatty acid levels; as DPA (docosapentanoic acid) and DHA levels increased, CRP levels deceased. These beneficially healthy oils are absent in the SAD in which the omega-6 to omega-3 ratio is as high as 25:1; the ratio should be around 3:1 to 2:1. The exact ratio is controversial. Omega-6 essential fatty acids promote inflammation and are needed when the body is traumatized and needs repair. **In other words we need some omega 6s but not nearly as much as in the SAD**. The two parent essential oils (PEOs) are linoleic acid and Alpha Linolenic acid. It is essential (no pun intended) to get these PEOs from unadulterated sources; plant and nut oils. The best dietary sources are; from flaxseeds and flaxseed oil, chia seeds, pumpkin seeds and pumpkin seed oil, and walnuts or walnut oil. Be aware, however, flaxseeds are phytoestrogens and mimic the effects of estrogen so I use chia seeds much more frequently. **Keep in mind you can go overboard eating too many omega-3 foods and taking too many omega-3 supplements. It is better to just decrease your omega-6 intake. This is easily accomplished if you just switch to a more Mediterranean or paleo type diet.**

Let's get back to my diet. For snacks, I consistently eat organic mixed nuts. I usually soak pecans, walnuts, and almonds for twenty minutes rinsing the lectins or proteins which annoy the intestines, then roast them on 200 degree heat for a few hours adding a generous amount of pink sea salt. I also add cashews, that do not need soaking, to roast. I avoid peanuts or peanut butter because according to many scientific studies they are susceptible to a mold that produces a mycotoxin called aflotoxin. Some other nutritious snacks are **Paleo People's Cacao mix** and **Veronica's Nut Mix**. These have only have 7 and 3 grams of sugar per serving, respectively, and both contain plenty of good fats. On some days I eat half of a low sugar protein bar with a handful of nuts. Before bed time I eat another apple with almond butter to get fiber, fat, and protein, keeping me satisfied until morning. **Remember too much sugar is metabolic poison to the body. You must not eat too much at one time or too often!**

To summarize: Many people do not like plain water and **never** drink it, opting instead for vitamin water, cow's milk, Starbuck's hot coffee/lattes, or iced coffee, soda, diet soda, or energy drinks. Any of these drinks containing caffeine as an ingredient is not a good choice and actually causes dehydration. Remember, it takes 32 ounces of water to make up for every 8 ounces of caffeine; a scary scenario even for the 4 cup and over per day coffee crowd. (I bet you will never forget this after my mentioning it

three or four times)! Although some studies have shown that one or two cups of coffee per day may limit one's chances of developing type 2 diabetes, so does just modifying the SAD. The caffeine speeds up the metabolism and burns more sugar. This probably is the reason for its diabetes prevention benefit. Remember, however, the caffeine high also has a low or a crash and makes the adrenal glands work overtime wearing them down. It is acceptable if you are a one to two cup per day coffee drinker as long as you drink one half of your bodyweight in pure water and an another liter per day to flush the kidneys and counteract the caffeine's dehydration effects. Also remember, soda has no nutritional benefit whatsoever; there are 10 teaspoons of sugar in each can, and it also contains phosphoric acid which interferes with the body's absorption of calcium possibly leading to osteoporosis, plaque buildup and cavities.
Researchers have found that those who began drinking soda when they were 12 years old had a 1.6 greater chance of becoming obese. Moreover, the GMO sweetener, high fructose corn syrup, contains traces of mercury- the most common toxic element in the body as you now know. For those of you that think diet soda is acceptable, think again. **Aspartame, the artificial sweetener in soda, is worse than table sugar;** this carcinogenic chemical has been linked to seizures, brain tumors, multiple sclerosis, emotional disorders and diabetes. And remember, it is banned in Europe.

Choosing to drink regular cow's milk is not worth the risk. In addition to containing the cow's growth hormones and anti-biotics, it also has harmful ingredients such GMO soybean and corn from the cow's diet. Remember the FDA allow something like 135 pustules on the cow's udders that supply the milk. If anyone can find a grass fed, drug fee cow's milk unadulterated or unpasteurized, it is more acceptable in moderation.

Sports drinks, like Monster, are extremely bad news and have been known to re-map the electrical system of the heart due to their incredibly high caffeine content, even resulting in some deaths. This is frightening to say the least! Like soda, they are also loaded with sugar which can lead to diabetes and obesity. It is one thing to drink a Gatorade after sweating like crazy while playing a sport. It is another to drink a case of Gatorade or Monster per week while just sitting around watching television or being sedentary.

You should drink one half of your bodyweight with good water. Avoid tap water containing chlorine, fluoride and other toxins. As I said previously, these compete with the iodine molecule essential to make thyroid hormone. The thyroid is the spark plug for the body's energy production. Buy mineral water and also avoid alkalized water because the stomach needs to be very acidic, and you are sabotaging your own digestion. **This also warrants repeating:** The body needs clean, clear water to filter 2000 liters of blood per day. The energy drinks and caffeinated, sugary drinks from Starbucks do not count as water. For variety and taste, put a lemon in your water; this also helps the body's detoxification ability. Sometimes I add a drop or two of dōTERRA brand Lemon or Lime essential oils to our water. Other times, I add a couple ounces of pure coconut water to a full glass or bottle of water. Avoid plastic bottles since the plastic leaches into the water; buy a glass or stainless steel water bottle. We use glass water bottles coated with rubber on the outside, making them safe if dropped. **Simply by drinking half of their bodyweight in ounces of water, many people will get rid of many of their symptoms because they have been in a chronically partially dehydrated state in which there is simply not enough water in the body to perform everyday essential tasks**. I know most people eating the SAD are prone to gallstones, even if they don't have a gallbladder in which the stones will be in the hepatic ducts of the liver. The normal bile which should flow freely becomes thick like sludge and then forms stones. A constant supply of good water will aid in preventing this from happening. Remember also, eating a lot of processed food and not drinking enough good water, this mixture will be too concentrated and thick, becoming harder to detoxify. Eventually it becomes kidney stones, another casualty of the lack of pure water.

I must turn to a great article that appeared in the journal, "Dynamic Chiropractic," written by Dr. David Seaman DABCN, who has diplomate status in nutrition, explaining in an excellent article that being in a state of ketosis, in which blood sugar averages between 65-80 mg/dL, is also an anti-inflammatory state. To really reach this point a person would only be able to consume about 50 grams or less of carbohydrates per day. Since it takes 4 calories to metabolize one gram of carbohydrate, this means a total of 200 calories per day coming from carbohydrates. I want the reader to see the irony in how blood sugar adversely affects the body and how taking medications just adds to the problem. (Don't be confused with ketoacidosis in which the Type 1 diabetic is prone to develop. They no longer produce the necessary insulin to prevent this from happening and must be more careful when following this type of eating plan. However, we have had several Type 1 diabetics, over the years, who have received great health benefits and weight loss by successfully completing our ketogenic T360 eating plan). **As I said and continued to say very often, Americans erroneously think that eating fat makes you fat and raises cholesterol levels; nothing can be further from the truth.** Now I will explain some science behind what happens at the enzymatic levels when a person eats carbohydrates versus fats. The Krebs cycle I discussed earlier is the process of how our bodies make energy from the food we eat. Keep in mind that the average American's diet consists of 40% refined carbohydrates; when ingested these excess carbohydrates are converted to pyruvate which is then converted into Acetyl-CoA and then finally to HMG (hydroxymethyglutaryl) Co-A. Cholesterol is formed when this HMG Co-A is converted into it by the enzyme HMG Co-A reductase. **I am telling you this because the mechanism of statin drugs is to block the action of this HMG Co-A reductase enzyme**. Now consider this for a moment. Americans have been frightened into not eating fat and cholesterol foods for fears of having a stroke or heart attack. So instead they have been eating more refined carbohydrates causing more insulin release. Guess what insulin stimulates? HMG Co-A reductase. Dr. Seaman states, "The outcome is that a high carbohydrate diet and its associated hyperinsulinemia (a lot of inulin in the bloodstream) equals hypercholesterolemia (a lot of cholesterol in the bloodstream) which means many people are put on statins for life." How is this for an exercise in futility? Dr. Seaman continues to say that when a person only eats a very low carbohydrate daily intake of less than 50 grams, the HGM Co-A reductase is not even turned on due to insulin not being stimulated. What happens is, since protein and fats are mostly being eaten, an enzyme called HMG Co-A lyse is turned on instead, leading to ketone body production feeding the brain and skeletal muscles. For those doubters who say that the ketone diet produces less energy than one from carbs, it is important to note that 100 grams of glucose will generate 8.7 kg of ATP (the fuel for our body produced by the Krebs cycle) while ketone bodies generate 9.4-10.5 kg of ATP. Furthermore, not only do ketone bodies produce more energy, but they also reduce oxidative stress or free radical damage, meaning a decrease in inflammation.

You are probably asking, "Who should be on this diet, should I?" Very convincing research is suggesting this diet is excellent for weight reduction and loss of appetite. Dr. Seaman writes, "This is extremely important for the overweight population, which generally has a strong appetite due to multiple metabolic abnormalities that enhance hunger." Strong evidence is also suggesting this diet for chronic disease processes such as diabetes, heart disease, and epilepsy, headaches, acne, Alzheimer's, Parkinson's, sleep disorders, autism, multiple sclerosis, cancer, and polycystic ovarian syndrome due to its desired anti-inflammatory state.

Dr. Seaman suggests that people, who are not trying to lose weight, eat about 100 or so grams of carbohydrates per day which equates to about 90 mg/dL of fasting glucose. If you have a chronic disease or are overweight, the ketogenic diet is the way to go. If you are thin and healthy, try to keep the refined carbohydrates down since much of the new research today is linking excess carbohydrate intake with future Alzheimer's and Parkinson's' diseases.

I must emphasize the importance of gluten free which is inherent in the paleo or autoimmune diet recommend by the Johnson board. It is not hard to do. Becky and I have been following it for almost six years now and both have noticed benefits. My facial and head rashes have ceased to occur as well as my severe pollen allergies. Becky had a constant thumping in her knees that she no longer has as well as a less bloated feeling after eating. From the genetic test findings I previously discussed, I am homozygous for the HLADQ2 SNP and Becky is heterozygous for the same gene. This means we both have a greater risk for having gluten intolerance or even Celiac's Disease (CD). We also both had symptoms of gluten intolerance. I try to correlate the diet with the gene results especially when there are overt symptoms. A biopsy is the gold standard to diagnose CD; however, the golden standard for gluten sensitivity is a three month modified elimination diet. I opted to just not eat it anymore after I learned that any wheat in this country is GMO and should be avoided.

For my auto-immune patients, I explain that the triggers for autoimmunity are usually gluten, dairy, and soy. The autoimmune diet I recommend is close to a pure paleo diet allowing no grains and avoidance of corn, rice, potato, and spelt. A patient should eat within 30 minutes of waking and then 4-6 small meals throughout the day to take the stress off the adrenal glands by keeping the blood sugar level steady. The goal with this is to heal the inflamed gut. Here are some cooking and eating tips to live by. Eat twice as many vegetables as fruits over the course of a day. Raw veggies are the best if you are trying to also lose weight. I always steam veggies so the vitamins are not cooked out of them. Cook in advance and prepare large batches of staples such as chicken, beef, and soups in single serving glass containers. To reheat food use a toaster oven or the stove top. I do not use a microwave oven. If you do, make sure you do not use plastic containers; they leach harmful chemicals when reheated.

In choosing proteins, select fish, wild game such as venison or buffalo, chicken, beef turkey, and pork. Wild caught fish is the best. Avoid farm raised fish and watch out for Frankenfish - genetically modified salmon. Predatory fish such as tuna and swordfish are loaded with mercury. Smoked salmon is acceptable. Try to vary the other meats frequently. Avoid Cured meats such as bacon, ham, and sausage which still can be eaten but not as an everyday staple. Look for organic without nitrates. "Al Fresco" is the brand of a great tasting chicken sausage that is gluten, dairy, and nitrate free and available at local grocers. Organic, grass fed, free range is always best.

Fresh veggies in multiple colors are essential. (I am not talking about corn, carrots, and peas either). You can get more vitamins and minerals with the different, bright colors. If a veggie is in a can, pass on it. Kale is a very important, versatile veggie that can be used in salads, soups, sautés and can even be dried and baked with olive oil and sea salt; baked kale tastes like potato chips. The key is making sure the leaves are dry when placed in the oven. You can even use it to make a green smoothie. (I have the recipe for mine at the end of the chapter). Don't be fooled by the smoothie mixtures in grocery stores loaded with sugar and all of the other unwanted ingredients. This way you can get the great nutrition from the raw dark leafy greens in your diet without even chewing them. The book called *Green For Life* contains many good green smoothie recipes. Moreover, cruciferous vegetables such as broccoli, cauliflower, brussel sprouts and cabbage are great sources of vitamins and minerals and also rich in Di-indolylymethane (DIM), which regulates hormones from all of the xenoestrogens (bad estrogens)/estrogen mimickers such as soy products. There are some who argue, from the results of animal studies, that since these cruciferous vegetables contain goitrogens which block the uptake of iodine, they will decrease the function of the thyroid gland and should be avoided by those with hypothyroid/Hashimoto's. Human studies, however, do not confirm this. Someone would have to consume 2 pounds per day of raw cruciferous vegetables to affect iodine production. If your thyroid problem is not from a deficiency in iodine, then this really doesn't apply because the anti-cancer properties of these veggies is too important to ignore. Xenostat from PRL is an excellent source of natural iodine and should be considered along with selenium to ensure proper iodine levels.

Sweet potatoes, purple sweet potatoes and purple potatoes are preferred, but skip the white ones and the white rice. Instead, buy long grain brown rice which requires 40 minutes to cook. If you have a rice cooker just add water and rice, turn it on and walk away. Quinoa is a nutty flavored corn based grain and is a substitute for rice and potatoes. (Remember however, corn is really considered a grain and not allowed on the true Paleo diet). Spaghetti squash can be substituted for pasta and is a staple in our house. There are also rice and corn based pastas and noodles that are very good choices.

For salads, choose dark greens like kale, spring mix or romaine and avoid the non-nutritious iceberg lettuce. If salad is the main meal, always include some protein such as grilled chicken, fish, beef, or shrimp. Nuts and fruits are very nutritious and also add great flavor in salads. Avoid most bottled dressings; they contain too many junk ingredients. I use Bragg's Vinaigrette and Ginger Sesame. It's also easy to just mix your own using olive oil, Bragg's apple cider vinegar and some seasonings.

Have about 2-3 servings of fruit per day. I eat a mixture of blueberries, strawberries, blackberries, and mangos with my morning buckwheat on exercise days, along with the banana in the green shake. Remember, I eat two apples a day, one at lunchtime and one with almond butter at bedtime. Keep in mind, however, fruit contains a lot of sugar even though it is natural; eat it only in small amounts. Diabetics must carefully monitor their fruit juice intake because it takes such a large quantity of fruit to fill an 8 ounce glass of juice: Moreover, the useful fiber is not included. **Make sure all fruit is organic, or else the pesticides add to the toxic soup.** Wash all fruit prior to eating it.

Nuts are a great snack, as you know, I eat them daily. Raw or roasted are good. Avoid salted nuts (unless sea salt) and those covered in honey. You can refer to the section on my diet, about four pages back, to see how I prepare the nuts.

Free range organic eggs, complete proteins, are especially good for us, including the yolks, and can be eaten at any meal. Remember, free range means that the chickens are not squeezed together in a pen and eating inferior grains consisting of canola oil and soybean meal. THE EGG SUBSTITUTES ARE LOADED WITH CHEMICALS; AVOID THEM.

Broths used to make soups should not contain any gluten or other thickening agents. Choose low sodium brands or use the water from blanching vegetables or cooking meats for your broth. You can also easily make your own highly nutritious **bone broth.** The Johnson forum just provided an interesting article by Charlotte Anderson in "Shape" magazine called, "8 Reasons To Bone Broth." I will list the eight benefits: 1). It heals your gut due to the gelatin which seals any leaks or holes in the intestine - a condition known as leaky gut, previously discussed. 2). Joint protection from the glucosamine and chondroitin sulfate. 3). The collagen helps a person look younger due to its plumping effect and also improves skin, hair and nails. 4). Sleeping ability is known to be better due to the glycine (a non-essential amino acid) which also improves memory. 5). It boosts your immune system due to its high concentration of minerals. A Harvard study that revealed some people suffering from auto-immune disorders not only experienced relief after drinking bone broth, but actually some achieved complete remission. 6). Strengthens bones due the magnesium, calcium, and phosphorus content. 7). Increased energy is noticed by bone broth drinkers although scientists are not sure of the mechanism. (I think it is simply due to the fact that the nutrition the bone broth reduces the burden/toxic load on the body so it can use that extra energy for some other necessary purpose). 8). It is very cheap to make and wisely uses those left over chicken and beef bones. Just cram the bones, herbs, and any veggies into a crock pot and put on low for 24-72 hours. After bringing to a boil, beef bones require more time simmering and chicken bones require less. Try to drink a mugful of either daily.

Cooking oils should primarily be olive and coconut oil. Coconut is preferred if you need higher temperatures. Stay away from the polyunsaturated junk oils like canola, vegetable oil, corn oil, and soybean oil. Real butter is good, but remember that margarine is one carbon away from plastic; AVOID ALL OF IT. A variety of herbs and spices greatly enhance almost all foods. Limit your table salt intake however; it is devoid of necessary minerals. Use pink sea salt liberally, one teaspoon per day helps to balance blood pressure not raise it.

Desserts are always a fun topic. Most people say they do not have a sweet tooth; I find that most people are kidding themselves. Some dessert suggestions are coconut ice cream, baked fruit, Paleo banana pancakes, and black bean brownies among many others available on assorted flour labels. (I will list the recipes shortly).

Snacks are the final topic for dietary advice. I sometimes eat hummus (a mixture of ground chick peas-garbanzo beans, tahini, lemon, garlic and sea salt) with some gluten free rice chips or veggies. You can purchase hummus or easily make your own with black, garbanzo, or northern white beans. Organic cashew, almond, pecan, walnut, and macadamia nut butters are a better selection than peanut butter because peanuts are grown in soil which naturally contains fungus and are vulnerable with their soft shell. These other nut butters can be spread on fruit, rice cakes, or gluten free bread and crackers for example. Protein bars are a good snack if you have nothing else handy, but they are hard to digest and sit in the stomach like a brick. Make sure they have a low sugar content and contain no soy. **Be sure to read the label carefully!**

I want to briefly discuss restaurant eating. It is not too hard to make good choices. Keep in mind that harmful canola oil is the oil most restaurants use because it is so cheap. When we eat out, I always bring a DHA capsule to counteract any inferior restaurant oil; the body recognizes the better oil and absorbs it, as I have already stated. More and more restaurants offer a gluten free menu today making it definitely easier to dine out.

Remember, however, if your goal is to lose weight, limit your visits to restaurants.

In cooking at home try to avoid Teflon frying pans, opting instead for cast iron which avoids any toxic fumes produced by non-stick pans, gives the benefit of a good source of iron in the diet from the pan which will boost your immune system, and can be used in the oven as well as on the stove top, even on high heat. Not only are they durable but they are also non-stick and can be easily cleaned.

A final important reminder about sugar. Considering that cancer rates are soaring today, the average person does not realize that cancer cells LOVE SUGAR and an anaerobic environment to thrive; this means they DO NOT LIKE OXYGEN. If you consume high amounts of sugar daily, you are really putting yourself at risk down the road. In fact, cancer cells consume 7.5 times more glucose than non-cancer cells. I also just recently mentioned the amino acid glutamine, which cancer cells need to synthesize more cells. Anyone who already has cancer should avoid a high SUGAR diet, and foods with glutamine such as RED MEAT, and DAIRY PRODUCTS (excluding cottage cheese), and WHEAT, and must increase the oxygen in the blood through exercise creating an aerobic environment. Therefore, you will short circuit the cancer cells from using glucose and multiplying. **You will decrease your chances of getting or surviving cancer, if you change your dietary habits**. Let's look at the hygiene products most people use that could definitely be harmful but also definitely easily replaced with some actually harmless. Just replace some of your products one at a time gradually so you do not become overwhelmed. You will definitely be taking the right step to enhance the health of you and your family. Every day, at the end of my shower, I moisturize with coconut oil, a great versatile oil having multiple properties; antibacterial, antiviral, anti-fungal and anti-protozoan. Very stable being saturated with hydrogens, it does not break down and go rancid once absorbed by the body and mixing with oxygen. This oil has also been found to decrease our body's need for Vitamin E indicating its anti-oxidant properties. Remember, **IF YOU RUB IT ON YOUR SKIN YOU SHOULD BE ABLE TO EAT IT.** Breathing it, rubbing it on, drinking it, or consuming it all have the same effects. If you moisturize with a chemical processed lotion, for example, would you then consider eating it? Those chemical laden lotions dry out your skin instead of moisturizing it. Also, most shaving creams for men and women contain too many harmful chemicals like Sodium lauryl sulfate, a drying agent and the main ingredient found in most cleansers requiring a lather including toothpaste, shampoo, shave creams and soaps, as I mentioned earlier. **This chemical is used in research experiments**

to remove the skin's lipid layer to determine how a much of an irritation the tested product will cause! Try to use a soap containing just basic ingredients, like one from dōTERRA, or the health food store, that can also be used by men and woman for shaving. I use dōTERRA's Grounding Blend essential oil as after shave to support a razor burn free face. Another product containing dangerous ingredients are Deodorants. Does it make any sense to rub the heavy metal aluminum under your arms where the sensitive lymph glands are? **This is really a very sensitive area.** I recommend Jungle Man deodorant containing only four ingredients to everyone; it can be purchases online at **junglemannaturals.com.** Look at the chemicals on the back of the deodorant you are currently using if you want to become shocked. Remember what I said in the FCT section; all of the toxic soup we are subjecting ourselves to daily, whether willingly or unknowingly, needs to be excreted from our body before it becomes embedded in the bone marrow or stored in fat where your immune cells cannot kill these toxins but will keep trying at your immune system's expense, resulting in an auto immune reaction.

Toothpaste selection is another challenge if you want a natural, chemical free one. A brand called "Kiss My Face" offers a non-fluoride version, which is the best I have found in a grocery store. However, it still contains sodium lauryl sarcosinate - a relative of sodium lauryl sulfate, also a foaming and drying agent. Beware of Tom's brand as it was bought out by Colgate and although it has several toothpastes that are SLS, many still contain titanium dioxide used as a whitening agent. A web store called Poofy Organics has a good chemical free toothpaste among other great products. There are many others free of either SLS or titanium dioxide but usually not both. We have been making our own toothpaste with my old standby coconut oil, baking soda, and essential oils. Use ½ cup of coconut oil, 2-3 tablespoons of baking soda, 1 tablespoon of xylitol, and ten drops of peppermint or spearmint essential oil.

Instead of those toxic petroleum products such as colognes and perfume, use essential oils. People always compliment my wife, who uses do-TERRA oils blends, that she smells so good. Women's Blend is the do-TERRA oil she often uses. She actually told me that just using the oil, Focus Blend, for her ADD tendencies serendipitously elicits a lot of male compliments on her choice of fragrance. Of course, they are shocked when she tells them she is just using essential oils and no perfume. For men there are several homemade recipes using the essential oils. For example, there is an earthy spice cologne using a mixture of clove, white fir, bergamot and lemon essential oils. (I have the exact recipe in the back of the book). Hunters use essential oils such as White Fir, Juniper Berry, and Douglas Fir to cover up their scent.

As I previously explained, commercial laundry detergents contain too many harmful chemicals. We have been using On guard laundry detergent from Do-Terra and love it; it is free of the harsh chemicals in regular detergents, containing a blend of only naturally derived surfactants, such as Propanediol, versus the petroleum based propylene glycol or glycerin. It also contains a bio-origin enzyme complex, and essential oil blend with 10ml of the do-TERRA essential oil in every bottle. Do-TERRA also has multiple cleaning recipe suggestions using their essential oils I have already listed many of these we use at home in the essential oils chapter.

Hair products such as shampoos and conditioners are my "forte"- just kidding of course, as I have had a shaved head since 1998. Additionally, there is an overabundance of make - up products on the market because woman especially demand a variety of distinct choices that the advertisers pander to. All of these products can be evaluated and rated by a phone app you can download called "Skin Deep." By scanning the product's bar code, the app will rate it from one to ten based on how many bad ingredients and carcinogens it contains. Many companies today, however, are starting to make their products paraben and phthalate free.

I must also address the medicine cabinet in most homes across America that contain a plethora of over the counter substances of which many could be replaced with do-TEERA essential oils. In fact, Becky actually has been teaching a class, "medicine cabinet makeover," where the average modern medicine cabinet contains about $812.79 worth of time consuming synthetic products that only treat symptoms, have side effects, an expiration date, and are time consuming to use. On the other hand, the Natural Solutions Kit from do-TERRRA is priced at $550 and offers all natural true healing products that have various positive effects, an extended shelf life and are both simple and efficient to use. For example, to support a urinary tract bacterial infection, a person can make a veggie capsule of Frankincense, Oregano and Protective Blend essential oils to be taken three times per day. A couple of drops of Cleansing Blend should also be rubbed in across the lower abdomen. This will support the immune system tremendously! **If a natural product works as well, or better, than a synthetic product, why wouldn't you use it?**

Dental fillings are a hot topic right now. The ADA (American Dental Association) dismisses the mercury filling controversy as totally inflated as I explained, insisting that silver amalgam fillings are very safe in spite of contrary data.? This includes Dr. Huggin's recommendations in, *It's All In*

Your Head, of both a hair and blood test for those with silver amalgams to identify whether they are irritating the body. Dr Huggins states, "It's not the presence of mercury that counts it's the body's reactivity to the mercury." The following are considered early warning signs or chemical indicators of mercury toxicity:

A white blood cell count above 7,500 or below 4,500.
Hematocrit above 50% or below 40%.
A Lymphocyte count above 2,800 or below 1,800.
Blood protein level above 7.5 grams per 100 milliliters or serum.
Blood triglycerides above 150.
BUN above 18% or below 12%.
Nickel found in hair analysis above 1.5 parts per million (ppm).
Hair mercury level above 1.5 ppm or below 0.4 ppm.
Hair aluminum level above 15ppm.
Hair manganese level below 0.3 ppm.

Here are some factors which may predispose people to problems with mercury fillings: The presence of root canal-treated teeth and the presence of both amalgam and gold. With two metals in your mouth, it is like a battery with your tongue as the ground. Mercury will leach out 80 times faster than normal!

As I previously recommended, in the FCT chapter, anyone choosing amalgam filling removal, should consult a Holistic or Homeopathic Mercury Free Dentist.

Finally, we must look at environmental toxins and what changes each of us could make to decrease our EMF exposure. I am aware that the close proximity of power lines to someone's house is beyond his control unless he considers moving, a choice not so affordable . However, there are PRL products mentioned previously such as Pyramids and Dragonite - a highly paramagnetic rock dust obtained from volcanic basalt, which can be used to limit the amount of man–made harmful EMF's from entering your property. You could also minimize other EMF exposures from cordless phones which emit a much larger EMF than even cell phones. If possible, get rid of any cordless phones; the base is the culprit. If you must use one at work, carry the phone in your office and make sure the base station is in the next room or as far away as possible. Furthermore, there is some new technology available for cordless phones called Dect. This base would only transmit when the phone is being used, cutting down on EMF's constant emissions.

Look around for a wired mouse and keyboard. I am using both plus a laptop writing this book. Wireless Wi-Fi and the mouse/keyboard all emit a lot of EMFs and could adversely affect you. Try to be about two to three feet away from your computer screen which should be LED not fluorescent backlit. This also applies to television screens. **Some researchers rate passive EMF radiation more harmful than cigarette smoking.** Try to sit at least 8-10 feet away from a big screen tv. At work and at home, replace all fluorescent light bulbs with mercury free ones; the mercury in these bulbs retards the excretion of the mercury in the body, one of the main focuses of FCT treatment. The mercury filled energy saving spiral bulbs should be replaced with halogen bulbs. Commercial fluorescent lights, such as those in office buildings, could be replaced with T8 mercury free bulbs. Often the ballast will also need to be replaced. I lucked out at my office as the T8 bulbs fit into the old ballasts.

Fortunately, there are certain filters called Stetzerizer which can be plugged into outlets to negate the negative effects of EMFs. The number of filters needed is based on the size of a house and the location of the main electrical box. The website for this is stetzerelectric.com.

There is another very effective, extensive system called Memon that as the company states, "neutralizes the negative influences of the information from electromagnetic fields, geographic fields of interference and harmful substances in water - all of which can exert negative influences on our bodies. They reduce the amount of dust in indoor environments." This system, however, is very expensive but works great. Some of my energy medicine practicing colleagues have this system installed in their house and office. This includes devices for cell phone protection also.

Where does a patient begin to apply this information, I have provided, to assess his own health while living in a toxic soup? I gave a lot of advice on what to eat and drink, what not to eat and drink, and what to environmentally change or avoid in your life. I tell my new patients in order to assess and treat their current health complaints/health challenges- or if no complaints, just to maintain overall health, we can offer these tests/treatments:

1). **Complete blood work analysis**
2). **Heavy Metal hair and urine analysis from Analytical Labs**
3). **A DNA test from 23andme**
4). **An FCT exam and treatment**
5). **A Zyto scan for essential oils (free to new patients)**
6). **A free PEMF treatment**

7). **Reiki**
8). **Infra-red Sauna**
9). **Aromatouch/Symphony of the Cells**

Note: *Any bloodwork done within the past year is good for me to evaluate without your having to get all new bloodwork.*

I correlate any testing results with the patients' history which more often than not includes a specific problem or symptom and then make the appropriate dietary, supplement, essential oil, environmental suggestions, and specific treatments such as FCT, PEMF, etc. For example, I have had numerous patients over the years, who discovered from functional analysis of bloodwork, that they had "high cholesterol" or a hypothyroid condition; conventional analysis did not reveal these. By correlating with QRA for the indicated supplementation and dietary modification, their next round of blood work, in about three months, was greatly improved. I have also had many patients with chronic low grade viral infections, even parasites that went under the radar through traditional blood work analysis only to also respond greatly to supplementation and dietary change. I am very excited to now offer these other great diagnostic and treatment methods. Another example, DNA testing, gives people that "oh" moment when they realize why they cannot get rid of a certain symptom or cannot eat a certain food without a negative reaction. Genes are permanent and can never be changed; however, we can alter whether they are turned on or off - their expression - (epigenetics) and the person's ability to greatly enhance the quality of his life.

Hair and/or urine heavy metal analysis offers another more complete picture of heavy metal toxicity as I previously explained, and reveals the extent of which metals are harbored in the patient's body, adversely affecting his health.

In FCT analysis we are checking the body for toxicity, which everybody has, in an objective fashion and then sending information to the body's bio-field, through energetic frequencies. These tell the body organs and tissues to release the toxins in a prioritized manner. **Often these toxins stored in the body are the main cause of all of the patient's symptoms.**

The following are some examples of cases that my colleagues and I have treated successfully using FCT over the past year: One woman was suffering from severe weekly migraine headaches and insomnia. An FCT exam revealed that she was very sensitive to EMFs. She was sleeping with her cell phone under her pillow and had it within inches from the body all day long. After the initial visit's remedy drops, she slept through the night for the first time in months. After six months of monthly treatments, her migraine headaches became a thing of the past. Another patient came in with shingles on his side after dealing with them off and on for a couple of months. The medical doctor told him there was nothing he could do except continue the meds he was already taking. He took the FCT remedy drops on Saturday morning and by Monday the shingles were 80% better. There was a middle aged woman who had chronic fatigue, swollen ankles, and depression. Her medical doctor told her she needed an anti-depressant; but she refused that advice. The third night after taking the FCT remedy drops, she passed two large kidney stones and reported that her leg swelling went down, and she felt like a new person. One of my colleagues had a stroke patient who suffered from stoke spasticity for the past 15 years. She had to have surgery to lengthen the tendons of the left arm so she could pull it away from her chest. After the surgery, she still could not get the arm away from her chest. Her left leg was also very spastic and her foot was curled up, forcing her to be in a wheelchair. She was also bedridden, due to depression and fear of being teased. After seeing one of my colleagues for 8 FCT visits, she said "I got my life back. I can walk with no problem and even dance!" **If the true cause or irritation is found, sometimes miraculous changes can happen.**

It is important to note that a session of <u>Reiki</u> with Becky is recommended to open the energy pathways and chakras which will enhance any other energy medicine therapy greatly!

The zyto scan also reads the body's biofeild and looks for homeostasis or balanced energy fields. Patients can try a few of the most suggested oils indicated to restore proper balance. We also perform Aromatouch and symphony of the cells therapy techniques in the office in which a few drops of many oils are combined and massaged into different parts of the body. These techniques, like FCT treatment, are attempting to balance the body through opening up detoxification pathways energetically which then tells the body to detox the actual substance. This should help support those with cardiovascular problems, chronic fatigue, lymphedema, digestive problems, and hormone imbalance, among other conditions.

We also recently added an IRS (Infra-red sauna) to our list of treatments enhancing detoxification. This can be used alone or to enhance our other energy techniques. Prior to the IRS, vibration therapy is used which warms up the muscles speeding up the metabolism.

The PEMF is such great a therapy that I cannot praise it highly enough. My colleagues and I on the Johnson board have had many cases with unbelievable results. A good example is, a male patient who had to urinate 4-5 times during the night for the past 10 years. After one PEMF treatment, he slept through the entire night for the first time in those 10 years. Following a series of PEMF treatments, he threw away his prostate medication. Moreover, I have many elderly patients, for example, who are able to stay on their feet for hours, have improved energy and enjoy an active life after PEMF treatments. These patients formerly spent most of their time sitting on chairs becoming drowsy and dozing.

Well, I guess that about wraps it up. It is time again to say goodbye for now. Remember, unless you live out in the boonies, like those in "Alaska: The Last Frontier" reality show, you are being pounded by air and water pollution, factory waste, dirty electricity cell phones, cell phone towers, wireless internet, and many other harmful wireless gadgets containing millions of harmful frequencies. Add to all of this the SAD and toxic sludge from industries including round-up farmers use on crops and round-up just about everybody uses on weeds at home. **We are under attack from environmental toxins; some you can see, taste and smell, but some, although silent, odorless and tasteless, are nevertheless just as deadly**.

Before reading this book, most of you probably read about nutrition and methods to improve your general health. Perhaps now, however, after having read the book, you can appreciate that there are more alternative choices in addition to the conventional ones to improve your metabolic and critical energetic health as well; all of the body's interdependent systems rely on a balanced biofeild. Remember the current food pyramid's recommendations of "whole grains," "milk," and unsaturated fats" for the past thirty years; how is that working for most people? Apparently, not so well; America's mortality rate even with its advanced technology is pathetic, to say the least. For the last time, I must state that the low fat, high carbohydrate diet, pushed hard in the seventies and even to this day, is a major contributor. **However, along with the erroneous dietary recommendations toxins need to be expelled and not stored in the body.** The energetic frequencies instruct the physical components of the body. By using energy techniques, such as FCT, we can offer the burdened body organ support so that heavy metal toxicity and other toxins can be more safely eliminated from the body than carelessly giving the patient a physical chelating agent **forcing detoxification without any necessary safety net**. For many patients who feel great and do not desire any testing, my advice is to **monitor your pH.** Just by doing this, you will become much healthier!

Living life is a little like playing Russian Roulette; nobody knows his toxic load threshold as it differs for each of us. But to stack the deck in our favor, or more aptly put, to further empty the chamber (of the loaded gun), I hope the suggestions I gave you in this book make a difference. Eating gluten free changed my family's and many of my patients' lives. I know many people do not like change that requires sacrifice; however, we cannot simply take drugs that cover up symptoms and go about living your life. REMEMBER THE SECTION ON GENES. RESEARCH NOW SHOWS THAT GENES ARE TURNED ON AND OFF BY ENVIORMENTAL INFLUENCE TO A FAR GREATER DEGREE THAN BY A PERSON'S GENETIC CODE. YOU NEED TO BEGIN EATING CERTAIN FOODS, USING CERTAIN HYGENE PRODUCTGS AND AVOIDING MANY OTHER FOODS, HYGEINE PRODUCTS AND EMF SOURCES YOU MAY BE ACCUSTOMED TO. **Energy medicine, existing for over three thousand years, has come full circle; it is the treatment of the future and here to stay!** Einstein said it so well, I will repeat it one more time: "EVERYTHING IS ENGERY AND THAT'S ALL THERE IS TO IT. MATCH THE FREQUENCY OF THE REALITY YOU WANT AND YOU CANNOT HELP BUT GET THAT REALITY. THIS IS NOT PHILOSOPHY. THIS IS PHYSICS." Take care of yourself and your family and please be aware of those measures you can take to reduce your toxic load; **YOUR HEATLH AND WELLNESS DEFINITELY DEPEND ON IT. SEIZE THE DAY!**

Wellness in a Toxic World

RECIPES:

PLEASE NOTE THAT ALL INGREDIENTS FOR ALL RECIPES ARE ORGANIC IF POSSIBLE.

My **GREEN SHAKE** recipe has the following ingredients:

- A bunch of leafy green vegetables such as swiss chard, collards, kale, etc.

- Bragg's apple cider vinegar

- coconut oil

- chia seeds

- protein powder such as whey or beef

- bananas or some other fruit

I make five servings at one time and freeze three servings so I only have to make them once per week.
I use 10 tablespoons of apple cider vinegar, 5 tablespoons of coconut oil, and 5 tablespoons of chia seeds. I mix the entire bunch of greens in and then throw in 5 scoops of 25-30 grams of protein powder followed by five bananas. I use water but almond milk or coconut milk could also be used.
Just remember to only use half as much fruit as veggies unless it is a post workout shake as in my case, in which you just exercised hard and your body needs the excess carbs/sugar. If you are not exercising before you drink it use more berries or fruits with a pit which have less sugar in them.

Please note that some of these recipes are paleo and some not due to the dairy. Coconut milk can usually be substituted for cream if gluten, dairy and soy free.

Beef Cabbage

1 Organic head of cabbage

1 medium onion diced

2 lbs. grass fed ground beef

3 cups of broth

1 can (32oz) organic fire roasted diced tomatoes

Salt and pepper to taste

******(Note all recipes calling for salt mean "sea salt.")

Brown beef in large pan, add onion, cabbage and broth. Cook on medium, stirring occasionally. When cabbage is cooked down and tender, add roasted tomatoes and salt and pepper. Simmer for 15 minutes and serve! (Alternatively, you can add all of the ingredients above into a crockpot and simmer for hours).

Banana Pancakes

1 ripe banana

2 eggs

Dash of cinnamon

Splash of vanilla extract

Mash banana, add eggs, cinnamon and vanilla and mix until smooth. Heat greased skillet and add small amounts of pancake mixture to skillet in small dollar size pancakes and cook until brown then flip. Options for toppings: fresh berries, Grade B Maple syrup, coconut syrup, coconut milk, raw honey.

Paleo Cauliflower Mac + Cheese

5 cups cauliflower

Sea salt + pepper to taste

1 cup coconut milk (rice or almond too)

½ cup broth

2 Tablespoons of coconut flour (or other)

1 egg beaten

2 cups grated cheddar cheese

Steam cauliflower and drain. Add to greased baking dish. In skillet heat coconut milk and salt + pepper on medium heat. Add broth while keep stirring then add flour while keep stirring. Bring to a bubble. Remove from heat and add whisked egg. Keep stirring. Pour over cauliflower and stir/mix then add cheese. Bake at 350 degrees for 35-40 minutes. Broil 3-5 minutes to a brown top.

Balsamic Chicken + Veggies

1 lb. boneless chicken breast

1lb. veggies such as asparagus or brussel sprouts

¼ cup of oil based Italian dressing

3 Tablespoons of balsamic vinegar

1 ½ Tablespoons of honey

1/8 teaspoon of red pepper flakes

Sea salt + pepper

Olive oil

Mix dressing, vinegar, honey, pepper flakes and set aside. Put olive oil in a skillet and add chicken plus salt and pepper. Cook for 10 minutes. Add ½ of dressing mix and cook another 10 minutes (until done). Remove chicken and set aside. Add veggies to pan salt and pepper to taste cooking until tender. Remove veggies and add to plates while putting chicken on top. With remaining dressing mix add to warm skillet and bring to a boil. When it thickens a little, add/drizzle on chicken /veggies. Amazing on top of polenta!

Slow Cooker Chicken Chili

1.5 lbs. boneless chicken breast

2 (14 0z.) cans fire roasted diced tomatoes

1 8 oz. can tomato sauce

1 14 oz. can corn rinsed and drained

1 14 oz. can black beans rinsed + drained

½ 8 0z. package of regular cream cheese, not low-fat or non-fat

1 cup chicken broth

1 red pepper finely chopped

1 jalapeno sliced and minced

½ yellow onion finely chopped

¾ Tablespoon of cumin

3 garlic cloves minced

1 ½ teaspoons of chili powder

1 teaspoon of oregano

Sea salt + pepper to taste

Place chicken in bottom of crockpot and add broth, tomatoes, beans, corn peppers, onion, jalapeno + garlic. Add seasonings and stir. Cook on high for 3 hours. Remove chicken and shred then return to crock pot and stir. Add cream cheese and stir. Cook another 20-30 minutes while stirring frequently until the cheese is melted. Garnish with cilantro, sour cream + tortilla chips.

Panko Breaded Chicken

Boneless, skinless chicken breast

Gluten free panko

Parmesan cheese

Garlic powder

Oregano

Eggs

Whisk egg in a bowl, mix panko cheese, garlic powder, oregano and put on plate. Cut chicken in tender sizes and dip in egg, then in cheese/panko spices mixture and place on a baking dish. Bake at 350 for 45-60 minutes or until brown.

Lasagna Stuffed Spaghetti Squash

2 small spaghetti squash cut in half + seeded

1 teaspoon of oil

1 lb. ground turkey

1 onion diced

2 cloves garlic, chopped

½ teaspoon of red pepper flakes

½ teaspoon of fennel seeds, crushed

1 (15 oz.) can crushed tomatoes

1 teaspoon of tomato paste (optional)

1 teaspoon of Italian seasoning or oregano

½ teaspoon of paprika

1 Tablespoon of balsamic vinegar

1 Tablespoon of basil, chopped/ 1 bay leaf

1 cup shredded mozzarella cheese

Brush inner flesh of squash with oil and season with sea salt + pepper. Roast (skin side up) the squash at 400 degrees for about 30 minutes or until tender. (For best results cut the squash perpendicularly or not long ways as it is easier to get the seeds out.) Meanwhile, cook turkey about 8-10 minutes and set aside. Heat oil in large pan on medium and add onion cooking for 5-7minutes. Add garlic, red pepper flakes + fennel and cook about a minute until fragrant. Add turkey, tomatoes, paste, oregano, bay leaf, paprika, balsamic vinegar, salt + pepper. Bring to a boil, reduce heat + simmer. Mix in basil then remove from heat. Fluff up inside of each squash, divide the mixture of the ricotta and basil between them followed by the sauce + cheese. Broil in the oven until cheese has melted and turned a light golden brown – about 2-3 minutes.

Sausage, Spinach, Feta Filling

Chicken sausage

1 cup feta cheese

1 package fresh spinach

I onion chopped

1 pepper chopped 1 package bella mushrooms

I can fire roasted tomatoes (diced)

Sauté sausage, onion, peppers and mushrooms in oil. When tender, add spinach and simmer. Add tomatoes + feta and mix together. Place in baking dish and bake 20 minutes or add to cooked spaghetti squash and bake for 20 minutes.

Chicken Piccata with Capers

1 lb. chicken breast

4 Teaspoons of Olive oil

1/3 stick butter

1 lemon

1 jar capers

1 clove garlic

Slice chicken thin and pound with a mallet until ¼" thick. Salt + pepper both sides. In large skillet, sauté butter, olive oil and garlic then add chicken. Brown both sides of chicken until cooked thoroughly. Remove from pan and set aside. In sauce pan, add lemon and capers. Continue to sauté olive oil, butter, lemon, capers, and chicken drippings - about 5 minutes on medium heat until mixture browns. Then pour over cooked chicken and serve.

Black Bean Brownies

1 (15 ounce can black beans, drained and rinsed

2 large eggs

¼ cup cocoa powder

2/3 cup honey

1/3 cup coconut oil

½ teaspoon of baking powder

Pinch of salt

4 drops of peppermint oil (optional)

¾ cups of unsweetened dark chocolate chips (optional)

Preheat oven to 350 degrees. Place all ingredients in a blender or food processor and blend until smooth. Pour batter into large bowl and stir in ¼ cup of unsweetened dark chocolate chips (optional). Bake for 30-35 minutes or until a toothpick inserted in the middle comes out clean. Let cool and cut into pieces. Store in refrigerator. You can boost the flavor of your brownies by adding other essential oils such as cinnamon, lavender, or wild orange - a different one each time you make them.

3 Minute Chocolate Paleo Mug Cake

3 teaspoons of almond meal

3 teaspoons of cocoa powder

2 teaspoons of honey

1 teaspoons of vanilla extract

1 egg

A few dashes of salt

5 dashes of cinnamon

*(Note: a variation is to use 2 teaspoons of cocoa powder with 1 teaspoon of sunflower seed butter).
I personally have gotten away from the microwave due to its harmful EMFs but will include this recipe as it seems to be a fan favorite.
Place all ingredients in a microwavable safe mug, stick in for three minutes and enjoy.

Roasted Veggies

Can use brussel sprouts , broccoli, asparagus or cauliflower.
Cut into manageable pieces. Add to zipper bag and toss with olive oil, salt + pepper. Lay flat on parchment paper lined baking sheet. Roast @ 400 degrees for 20-30 minutes or until browned. Note: Cook these until they almost appear burned. Most people undercook these and they remain hard. They will loosen up considerably when cook longer.

Here is the recipe for Earthy Spice I discussed earlier. It can replace harmful petroleum based colognes:

Earthy Spice Cologne

10 drops Clove essential oil

20 drops White Fir essential oil

40 drops Bergamot essential oil

5 drops Lemon essential oil

280 drops do-TERRA Fractionated Coconut Oil

There are more of these available at www.dōTERRAeveryday.com

I talked a lot about gluten free in my first book and some in this one as well so I added the following handout a Johnson Forum doctor put together. (I do not know his name to thank him.) I give this to patients who wish to begin following the gluten free lifestyle. Remember, going gluten free is also reducing your toxic chemical load due to the fact that the number one xenobiotic, (a chemical compound such as a drug, pesticide, or carcinogen foreign to a living organism) the weed killer round-up, is sprayed on wheat! Here it is:

Getting Started on a Gluten Free Diet
(Beginning your gluten-free journey toward a healthier life!)

What Is Gluten?

Gluten is a sticky protein found in certain grains such as wheat, barley, rye, spelt and Kamut. Since it is so sticky, it acts like a glue to bind ingredients together. Gluten holds together the flour which makes bread. Gluten stops sauces, gravies, and soups from curdling and gives a smooth texture to cheese spread and dips, dressings, margarines, sweets, canned meats, mustard, and almost all packaged and processed foods. It has therefore been in the interest of the manufacturers to use it extensively and in the interest of the growers to increase the gluten content of grains.

LET'S START WITH....
WHAT YOU CAN EAT!

Lots of things! While it is true that a lot of food will now be off limits, it is also true that there is a lot of food in the world~ and many things are still perfectly safe to eat! Getting back to basics is a good way to start.

You can still eat:
Fruits
Berries
Nuts and Seeds
Vegetables
Meat
Poultry
Fish
Eggs
Milk, Cheese, and Yogurt (if not casein or lactose intolerant)
Potatoes
Rice

Please rest assured that you can buy or make your own gluten free baked goods~ bread, cakes, cookies, muffins, and more!

There are several brands of gluten free beer on the market now, and an endless supply of gluten free snack foods like popcorn, peanuts, gf pretzels, gf crackers, corn chips, etc. Many restaurants offer gluten free menus.

It really is best to begin with a basic whole foods diet and it is also important to focus on what you CAN HAVE rather than dwell on what you can't have. It's that whole positive thinking thing.

Whole grains like quinoa, buckwheat, and amaranth are acceptable on the diet as long as you are not sensitive to them.. It can be fun to explore new foods, and you may find with the new focus on food you will actually increase the variety of healthy foods in your diet; most of us do!

"Back to basics" eating is just easier while on the gluten free diet learning curve. Reading labels at the grocery store can be daunting in the beginning. That gets easier over time as you eventually learn which foods and ingredients are acceptable.

You will eventually get back to a regular shopping list~ it will just be a little different than it was before. Eating unadulterated whole foods over processed foods really cuts down on label reading.... a big help when beginning this overwhelming task of re-evaluating everything you eat!

Whole foods, unprocessed foods, are just healthier for you all the way around, and are easier on your intestinal system while it is healing. You will be reducing the risk of inadvertent gluten errors by avoiding processed foods, and giving your body a better chance to heal quickly.

It is not uncommon for those with gluten sensitivity or celiac disease to suffer from other food intolerances as well. In fact, studies tell us up to 50% of those with celiac disease or gluten sensitivity also have problems with cow's milk. Corn and soy sensitivity are commonly a problem as well.

Sticking to whole foods, and keeping a food and symptom journal, can help to identify additional sensitivities if you continue to have symptoms. Many people find they do much better without any grains at all in their diet.

Do I Have To Buy Expensive Specialty Foods?

No! In fact, you can live quite nicely and healthfully without any of the specialty food products. Many opt to eat only naturally gluten free whole foods and find this simple way of eating very satisfying.

There are also many mainstream processed foods that are gluten free and safe for you to eat. Some mainstream products are even beginning to clearly label products as gluten free... which makes our job of label reading a lot easier.

Allergy and Contains Statements on products are also very helpful, but beware because they won't necessarily include barley or rye ingredients. Wheat is one of the eight major allergens covered under labeling laws. When you see wheat in a Contains: statement, or highlighted in the ingredient list, it shortens the label reading task as you quickly return the product to its store shelf.

Specially Foods Galore If You Still Want Them

There are many specialty gluten free foods on the market and the market is growing like wild fire. More products are making their way to your very own local grocery store... be sure to check the health and specialty aisles! Most health food stores will carry a wide variety of gluten free products.

The GF Mall is a one stop directory of websites offering foods in the gluten free specialty market. There is a searchable data base of GF products at GF Overflow.

One caution about specialty foods... though. They are not necessarily HEALTHY foods. Once you begin to read labels of everything you eat, out of necessity, you will gain an acute awareness of exactly what you are eating. Many of us end up cleaning up our diets overall and doing without much of the processed foods, but for some of us who still like to splurge on occasion with a little junk food... it is still all available!
No shortages there....

Can I Make My Own Baked Goods?

Yes, you can!

It is simple to purchase various gluten free flours and make your own baked goods. You can buy pre-blended gluten free flours, or blend your own... usually a combination of rice flour, tapioca flour, and potato starch flour. The healthiest flours to bake with are almond flour and coconut flour and recipes can be found on elanaspantry.com. There are many gluten free recipe books on the market if you look for them. According to Amazon.com there are 276 of them, and counting!

Online and local support groups are also very helpful in supplying gluten free recipes and baking tips. And don't throw away your old cook books either! It is very simple to convert most recipes, especially when cooking, but even when baking. You can make a mean Toll House cookie right off the Nestle package, with a simple substitution of gluten free flour, and an added teaspoon of xanthan gum or guar gum.

And What You Can't Eat….

Bread, cakes, pies, cookies, pasta, candy, or any other product that uses wheat, rye, or barley needs to be avoided. Don't be fooled... white bread is indeed made with wheat flour!

Avoid anything made with:

Wheat - *including einkorn, emmer, spelt, Kamut, wheat starch, wheat bran, wheat germ, cracked wheat, hydrolyzed wheat protein*
Bromated flour
Durum flour
Enriched flour
Farina Graham flour
Phosphated flour
Plain flour Self-rising flour
Semolina
White flour
Barley
Couscous
Rye & Triticale - *a cross between wheat and rye*

Gluten may also be found in other processed foods you might not suspect, so it is important to read labels carefully. You'll need to ask questions when eating at restaurants, and at the homes of family and friends. It is generally possible to find gluten free brands of many of these items, but you must be especially cautious about the following items~ and verify!

Bouillon cubes
Brown rice syrup
Chips/potato chips
Candy (including licorice!) & chewing gum
Cold cuts, hot dogs, salami, sausage

Communion wafer
French fries, fryer oil may be contaminated or if they are breaded
Glazed Hams - glaze or injections
Gravy – all-purpose flour is usually the thickener
Imitation fish – additives and fillers
Marinated Meats – the marinade
Matzo
Rice mixes – the seasoning packet
Sauces
Seasonings
Seasoned tortilla chips, French fries, potato chips
Self-basting turkey
Soups
Soy sauce- substitute with Tamari sauce

Important: Reading Labels

Reading labels must become a new part of everyday life unless you remove *all* processed foods from your diet. We need to read labels at the grocery store, and reread them again before opening a can, box or package at home. And because ingredients often change~ we must read labels over and over and over again, even when purchasing products we think we "know" are safe.

Being a member of a gluten sensitivity or celiac disease community, locally or online, can be immensely helpful when starting out on a gluten free diet. There are a lot "tricks to the trade"... and generally, others who have been doing this for years can tell you exactly which brands are currently safe. Local support groups are also very helpful, and will be able to tell you the best gluten free shopping spots, and gluten free restaurants in the area.

What About Oats?

Some oats may be contaminated with gluten because of cross contamination in the fields or during processing. Consequently, *whether or not oats are safe to eat remains a controversial subject.* The majority of research on the subject indicates that oats are safe for people with gluten sensitivity or celiac disease, but it remains in question. Some people may also have a separate sensitivity to oats.

If you do choose to include oats in your diet, look for a brand which has gluten free certification. It may be wise to eliminate them completely from your diet for the first several months, and add them back only if all is

well, and then do so with caution.
Bob's Red Mill GLUTEN FREE Oats, Glutenfreeoats.com
Creamhill Estates, Only Oats

How Strict Do I Need To Be?

You need to be very strict~ 100% diligent about removing all gluten from your diet. A tiny little bit, even in the form of cross contamination, can do damage if it occurs often enough~ preventing your intestines from healing, and keeping your immune system producing destructive antibodies.

One of the best analogies I've heard is of comparing damaged intestinal villi to a skinned knee. If you skin your knee, and then keep falling down every couple of days and re-scraping it, it will never heal. Cross contamination and gluten errors are like falling down and re-scraping your knee. You'll never get better if you keep falling.

Some people may not react symptomatically to gluten errors, but that doesn't mean the infractions aren't doing any damage. Repeated errors will keep those antibodies in production and working against you, even if you aren't noticing any symptoms on the 'outside'.
If you are auto-immune, eating gluten, is like THROWING GAS ON A FIRE!

CROSS CONTAMINATION

Beyond checking labels for safe ingredients, those on a gluten free diet have to worry about cross contamination that can occur in the home, school, workplace, manufacturing environments, etc. Rather than reinvent the wheel, here are some links to things you need to think about.

Cross Contamination Potential Issues by Mireille
http://forums.delphiforums.com/n/mb/message.asp?webtag=celiac&msg=32462.1 (may enter as guest)
How to Make Your Home Gluten Free
by Children's Hospital Boston

Cross- Reactive Foods & Foods You Might Be Sensitive To

There are 13 foods commonly cross-reactive with gluten. They are: cow's milk, alpha-casein and beta-casein, caseomorphin, milk butyrophin, American cheese, milk chocolate, rye, barley, spelt, Kamut (polish wheat), yeast oats, and coffee. Cross reactive means the amino acid sequences are so similar that the immune system can react as if you are still eating gluten.

There are 11 foods not cross-reactive, but patients on a gluten-free diet are frequently sensitive to and they are: sesame, hemp, buckwheat, sorghum, millet amaranth, quinoa, tapioca, corn, rice and potato (not sweet potato). An accurate test at our office is available for the above.

Paleolithic Diet

Some people with gluten sensitivity find they do better with no grains at all, and opt to follow a Paleolithic diet, which is not only gluten free, but grain free, casein free and legume free. To learn more:
www.thepaleodiet.com
www.paleofoodmall.com

List of Gluten Derivatives

Alcohol made from grains: beer, whisky, vodka (unless potato based), scotch: most liquors (However the distillation process nullifies any gluten threat to those gluten sensitive. This may not be true with those with known Celiac's or some others.)
Batter-coated foods
Biscotti
Bran
Canned meat containing preservatives
Canned vegetables (unless canned in water only)
Caramel (made and imported from countries other than the US and Canada)
Chewing gum
Curry powder
French fries (may be fried in the same oil as bread products)
Fruit drinks
Horseradish sauces
Hydrolyzed vegetable protein (may be made from wheat)
Imitation seafood (usually made with a starch binder made of wheat)
Instant hot drinks-coffee, tea, hot chocolate
Ketchup – unless stated "gluten-free"
Modified food starch
Rice syrup (may contain barley malt)
Salad dressings –avoid commercial varieties unless noted "gluten-free"
Soups-most commercially made canned or frozen soups
Soy sauce and most other Chinese sauces, except for Tamari wheat free sauce

White pepper
Malt
Veined cheeses (may be created with molds that could be of bread origin)
Bullion cubes or powder (artificial color)
Mustards – unless stated "gluten-free"
Margarines
Sauces
Sausages
Starch
Sweets, such as cakes, pastries, cookies , candies, muffins, chocolate unless noted "gluten free" on label
MSG (Monosodium Glutamate) – flavor enhancers
Glutamic Acid & Monopotassium Glutamate– flavor enhancers

Some Suggestions:
- Buy good ingredients.
- Buy organic whenever possible especially produce on the "The Dirty Dozen" list
- Limit pesticide exposure.
- Don't purchase packaged, frozen, or canned foods except for tuna, some beans and coconut milk.
- Always eat before you go to a party so you do not experience hunger pangs.
- Always carry a snack with you when you go out in case your plans change and you cannot find anything to eat.
- Be cautious to accept someone's word that the food they are offering is gluten-free unless you are really sure.
- Do not be tempted just because you are feeling better, to assume you are cured! Be warned – if your body has just started to recover, it will be even more sensitive to the food and the reaction will be dramatic.

Transitioning to a Gluten Free Life

Get educated. There is on-line help, books, support groups, our office, etc. You are not alone!
Clean your kitchen. If the whole family is going gluten free, give away your non gluten-free food. If it is only part of your family, get out labels and start marking what is gluten- free.
Learn how to shop and where to shop. Start reading labels and looking for hidden sources of gluten in processed foods.
Discuss your needs with your family and friends. Notify them that you

are living gluten-free. Let them know so when you plan to get together there are gluten-free options.

Transition away from your normal day-to-day diet.

Be a conscious eater! Think about your food choices and be aware that these decisions are leading you toward a healthier life. (Many individuals with a gluten intolerance may have reactions to other grains as well, so be aware of such a possibility.)

Go to restaurants that provide gluten-free options. Always tell the waiter that you are gluten-free so he can notify the chef. Many restaurants will customize a dish for you if they know. And be aware that when eating at restaurants that do not have gluten-free menus, there are many foods contrary to your expectations that may contain gluten. Be sure to check with your server and if they don't know, have them ask the chef. Your health is important!

Here are some snack ideas I got from Dr. Corey King. Little snacks for on the go:

- Pea Protein shake. Mix with water, coconut milk or coconut water.
- Cucumbers with olive oil, lemon salt and pepper dressing.
- Dill Pickles
- Apple, peach, nectarine, cherries
- Cucumbers and Guacamole
- Epic Protein Bar (www.epicbar.com)
- Chicken Salad (a whole chicken with diced celery and onion, dill relish, Dijon mustard, and organic mayonnaise. Salt and pepper to taste.
- Lettuce Wraps (Some type of meat, avocado wrapped up in lettuce and dipped in olive oil and vinegar dressing or hummus)
- Hummus with veggies
- Coconut yoghurt or kefir with fruit

For breakfast ideas:
- Chicken /Tukey sausage (Applegate is a great brand)
- Salmon for breakfast, with onions and/or capers
- Eggs any style
- Some sweet potato hash with onions, some cinnamon sautéed with coconut oil, can be made in a big batch ahead of time and reheated.
- Turkey egg cup. Take a slice of turkey and break an egg on top then bake at 350 for 10-15 minutes. You can top with avocado, sea salt and cracked pepper.

- Shredded sweet potato egg cups. Take shredded sweet potatoes and spritz with olive oil, salt and pepper to taste. Bake for 10-15 minutes at 350 degrees then pour egg on and bake again for 10-15 minutes then top with avocado and bacon.

Enjoy this journey to a healthier life!

REFERENCES

1. GILDEA, MARTIN DC, CFMP *HEALTH:* "A COMMON SENSIBLE APPROACH "(CREATE SPACE 2014) PG 52
2. MILHAM, SAMUEL MD, MPH "DIRTY ELECTRICITY "(2ND EDITION, I UNIVERSE 2012) PGS. 69-71
3. HUGGINS, HAL DMD "IT'S ALL IN YOUR HEAD" (AVERY PUBLISHING) PAGE 11
4. MILLER, NEIL & GOLDMAN, GARY "HUMAN EXPERIMENTAL TOXICOLOGY" 2011 SEPTEMBER 30(9): 1420-1428
5. MEGAN BROOKS *WEB MD* AUGUST 5, 2014
6. GILDEA, MARTIN DC. CFMP HEALTH: "A COMMON SENSIBLE APPROACH" (CREATE SPACE 2014) PG 60
7. KHARRAZIAN, DATIS DC, MS "WHY DO I STILL HAVE THYROID SYMTOMS? (M&J NEW YORK 2010) PGS 68-70
8. WEATHERBY, DICKEN ND AND FERGUSON, SCOTT ND BLOOD CHEMISTRY AND CBC ANALYSIS" (BEAR MOUNTAIN PUBLISHING 2002)PGS. 10-11
9. TENNENT, JERRY MD " HEALING IS VOLTAGE" (TENNENT PUBLISHING 2013)PGS. 216,221,329
10. WEATHERBY, DICKEN ND AND FERGUSON, SCOTT ND "BLOOD CHEMISTRY AND ANALYSIS" (BEAR MOUNTAIN PUBLISHING 2002 PG17
11. WEATHERBY, DICKEN ND AND FERGUSON, SCOTT ND "BLOOD CHEMISTRY AND NALYSIS " (BEAR MOUNTAIN PUBLISHING 2002 PG 5
12. WAYNE L SODANO DC, DABCI & RON GRISANTI DC, DABCO, MS "FUNCTIONAL DIAGNOSTIC MEDICINE TRAINING AND PROGRAM/INSIDER'S GUIDE MOD1 LESSON 7 BLOOD CHEMISTR & CBC ANALYSIS (FUNCTIONAL MEDICINE UNIVERSITY PUBLISHING PAGE 16
13. WEATHERBY, DICKEN ND AND FERGUSON, SCOTT ND "BLOOD CHEMISTRY AND ANALYSIS " (BEAR MOUNTAIN PUBLISHING) 2002 PG 181

14   OWEN M RENNERT AND WAI-LEE CHAN, "METABOLISM OF TRACE METALS IN MAN (CRC PRESS, INC 1984) VOL 1 PGE 102

15   ANTHONY COLPO "THE GREAT CHOLESTEROL CON" (LULU PUBLISHING 2006) **PAGES** 150-158

16   JOANNE GUTHRIE AND BIING-HWAN LIN (USDA RESEARCH SERVICE MAY 5, 2014) "HEALTHY VEGETABLES UNDERMINED BY THE COMPANY THEY KEEP"

17   THE US DEPARTMENT OF AGRICULTURE AND HEALTH AND HUMAN SERVICES "DIETARY GUIDELINES FOR AMERICANS 2010" PAGE X

18   DAVID BROWNSTEIN MD "SALT YOIUR WAY BACK TO HEALTH' (MEDICAL ALTENATIVES PRESS) PAGES 25-28,44-47.

19   "PHYSIOPATHOLOGICAL EFFECTS OF RAPESEED OIL: A REVIEW, "BORG, K. ACTA MED SCAND SUPPL (1975), 585: 5-13 ISSN: 0365-463X

20   JERRY TENNANT, MD, MD(H), PSC,D "HEALING IS VOLTAGE" (TENNANT INSTITUTE) PAGES 214-239

21   JAMA. 1984 JAN 20;251 (3):365-74

22   ALEXSANDRA OSSOLA "POPULAR SCIENCE" 2015 JUNE 17

23   GILDEA, MARTIN S DC "HEALTH: A COMMON "SENSIBLE" APPROACH" (CREATE SPACE PUBLISHING) PAGES 18-23

24   REX AND ROBERT JAMES " ESSENTIALS OF THE EARTH" (ESSENTIAL OILS BOOK) PAGES 6-7

25   AROMA TOOLS "MODERN ESSENTIALS" (AROMA TOOLS PUBLISHING) PAGES 11-13

26   VALERIE ANN WORWOOD"THE COMPLETE BOOK OF ESSENTIAL OILS & AROMATTHERAPY" (NEW WORLD LIBRARY) PAGE 8

27   VALERIE ANN WORWOOD "THE COMPLETE BOOK OF ESSENTIAL OILS & AROMATHERAPY" (NEW WORLD LIBRARY) PAGE 9

28. AROMA TOOLS " MODERN ESSENTIAL" (AROMA TOOLS PUBLISHING) PAGES 48-49
29. AROMA TOOLS "MODERN ESSENTIALS"(AROMA TOOLS PUBLISHING) PAGES 16-19
30. HS BURR "THE FIELDS OF LIFE" (NEW YORK: BALLATINE BOOKS PUBLISHING) PAGES 10-15
31. RICHARD GERBER MD "VIBRATIONAL MEDICINE" (BEAR AND COMPANY ROCHESTERVERMONT) PAGES 40-45
32. W TILLER "PRESENT SCIENTIFIC UNDERSTANDING OF THE KIRLIAN DISCHARGE PROCESS" (PSYCHOEREGETIC SYSTEMS, VOL 3, NOS 1-4 1979
33. ROBERT O BECKER, MD AND GARY SELDEN "THE BODY ELECTRIC" (NEW YORK MARROWPUBLISHING) 1985 PAGES 80-104
34. SMALLIKARJUN "KIRLIAN PHOOGRAPHY IN CANCER DIAGNOSIS" OSTEOPATHIC PHYSICIAN, VL 45 NO.. 5 1978 PAGES 24-27
35. B GRIGGS " GREEN PHARMACY: A HISTORY OF HERBAL MEDICINE (NEW YORK VIKINGPRESS) 1981 PAGES
36. TREVOR SMITH MD "HOMEOPATHIC MEDICINE" (HEALING ARTS PRESS) 1984 PAGE 15
37. CW LEADBEATER "THE CHAKRAS" (THEOSOPHICAL PUBLISHING HOUSE) 1977 PAGES 5-10
38. RICHARD GERBER MD "VIBRATIONAL MEDICNE (BEAR AND COMPANY PUBLISHING) 2001 PAGES 143-145
39. RICHARD GERBER MD "VIBRATIONAL MEDICNE (BEAR AND COMPANY PUBLISHING) 2001 PAGES 513-515
40. W TILLER "THE POSITIVE AND NEGATIVE SPACE/TIME FRAMES AS CONJUGATE SYSTEMS" IN FUTURE SCIENCE, ED. WHITE AND KRIPPERNER, (GARDEN CITY, NY DOUBLEDAY & CO, INC PUBLISHING)1977 PAGES 257-275
41. GERBER, RICHARD MD " VIBRATIONAL MEDICINE" (BEAR AND COMPANY

PUBLISHING) 2001 PAGES 179-181
42. YURKOVSKY, SAVELY MD "THE POWER OF DIGITAL MEDICINE " (SCIENCE OF MEDICINE PUBLISHING) 2003 PAGE 5
43. MARTIN S GILDEA DC CFMP HEALTH : A COMMON "SENSIBLE" APPROACH (CREATE SPACE PUBLISHING) 2014 PAGE 64
44. HAL HUGGINS MD "ITS ALL IN YOUR HEAD"(AVERY PUBLISHING) 1993 PAGES 6-11
45. BYRANT A MYERS "PEMF THE FIFTH ELEMENT OF HEALTH" (BALBOA PRESS) PAGES 138-150
46. **SUBTLE ENERGIES & ENERGY MEDICINE (2007, VOLUMBE 18,#2, PAGES 55-61)**
47. JERRY TENNANT, MD "HEALING IS VOLTAGE" (TENNANT PUBLISHING) PAGES 89-164
48. SHERMAN R ET.A.L. "ORTHOPEDIC SURGERY SERVICE" MADIGAN ARMY MEDICAL CENTER, TACOMA WA, USA)
49. JORGENSEN W ET AL "INTERNATIONAL PAIN RESEARCH INSTITUTE " LOS ANGELES, CA
50. KAAN UZUNCA, MURAT BIRTANE AND NURETTIN TASEKIN "THE CLINICAL RHEUMATOLOGY JOURNAL, VOLUME 26-1 JANUARY 2007 (SPRINGER LONDON)
51. MURRAY J. ET.AL. "MODULATION OF COLLAGEN P RODUCTION IN CULTURED FIRBROBLASTS BY A LOW-FREQUENCY PULSED MAGNETIC FIELD" (BIOCHIM BIOPHYS ACTA)
52. MARKS RA. "SPINE FUSION FOR DISCOGENIC LOW BACK PAIN:OUTCOME IN PATIENTS TREATED WITH OR WITHOUT PULSED ELECTROMAGNETIC FIELD STIMULATION"(RICHARDSON ORTHOPEDIC SURGERY, TX)
53. CONNER, KEVIN DC "STOP FIGHTING CANCER & START TREATING THE CAUSE (UPPER ROOM WELLNESS) PAGES 95-107
54. KHARRAZIAN, DATIS DHSC, DC, MS "WHY DO I STILL HAVE THYROID SYMPTOMS WHEN MY LAB TESTS ARE NORMAL" (MORGAN JAMES PUBLISHING) 2010 PAGES 40-59
55. SEAMAN, DAVID DC,MS, DABCN "GETTING TO KETOSIS-AN ANTI-INFLAMMATORY STATE" (DYNAMIC CHIROPRACTOR) FEB 2014